The
Ehlers-Danlos / Arachnoiditis
Connection

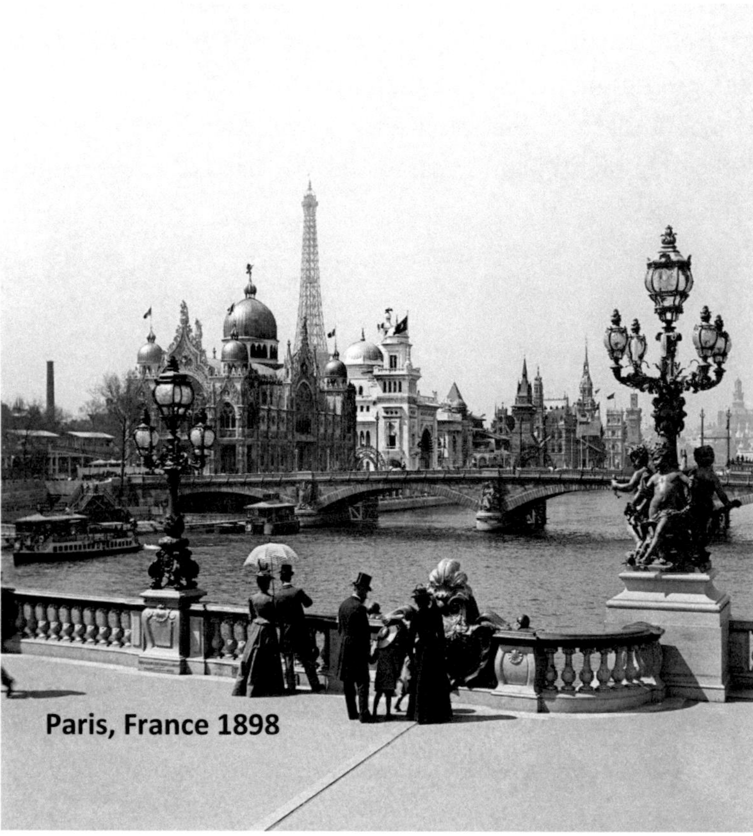

Forest Tennant, DrPH, MPH, MD

Picture on Cover

In 1899 Dr. Lauritz Edward Ehlers, a Danish dermatologist presented a law student with lax skin, loose joints, and a tendency to develop hematomas in the skin to the French Dermatologic Society. This was the first medical recognition of an inherited collagen deficiency, connective tissue disease. This first case presented in Paris is now recognized with Ehlers being the first name in Ehlers-Danlos Syndrome. Interestingly the second case of this disease was also presented in Paris in 1908 by Dr. Henri Danlos whose name is second in the name of the disease.

The
Ehlers-Danlos / Arachnoiditis Connection

By

Forest Tennant, DrPH, MPH, MD

Published by the
Tennant Foundation
West Covina, California

SPONSORS OF THIS BOOK
Tennant Foundation
336-338 S. Glendora Ave.
West Covina, CA 91790-3043
Ph: 626-716-2689
Fax: 626-919-7497
Email: tennantfoundation92@gmail.com

ISBN: 9781955934374
Library of Congress Control Number: 2024911409

U.S. trade bookstores and wholesalers: Please contact. Nancy Kriskovich
Tel: (406)249-2002; or
email snkriskovich@gmail.com

All proceeds from the sale of this book will go to the Medical Study and Education Projects sponsored by the

Tennant Foundation
336-338 S. Glendora Ave.
West Covina, CA 91790-3043
Ph: 626-716-2689
Fax: 626-919-7497
Email: tennantfoundation92@gmail.com

Acknowledgements
Medical Director
Martin J. Porcelli, DO, MPHE, PhD

Research and Reviews
Ingrid Hollis

Publication Development
Rebecca Cholcher-Marino
Nancy Kriskovich

Dedication:

To Donna Corley who has inspired me and others to research and help people with EDS, AA, and Tarlov cysts. Donna pioneered social groups for both arachnoiditis and Tarlov cysts. Due to her single efforts, thousands have found some relief, comfort, and quality of life.

Table of Contents

AUTHORS NOTES

This book has been written to call attention to the connection of Ehlers-Danlos Syndromes (EDS) and adhesive arachnoiditis (AA). The combination of these two diseases is a medical tragedy of great misery, suffering, and a shortened life. Persons with this dual disease combination need to be recognized at the earliest date possible so they can hopefully stop the pathologic progression of their plight and have some quality of life. This dual disease combination can probably be prevented or at least ameliorated if all concerned parties have a basic understanding of how the two diseases become connected.

The discovery of this disease combination has been unexpected. It grew out of my Foundation's studies on arachnoiditis and intractable pain. A major goal of our research has been to determine the causes of AA so it can be prevented. In our efforts we have reviewed and maintain an inventory of over 1000 magnetic resonance imaging (MRI) studies of adhesive arachnoiditis cases. Much to our surprise we have found that at least 30-50% of the cases have EDS. Based on what I have learned, every person with EDS is at risk of developing AA. I also now believe that AA can be prevented in essentially all cases, and this is a major motivation for writing this book.

PROLOGUE

At the start of this century, both EDS and AA were considered rare diseases. In a relatively short time both diseases have emerged as clinical entities that are sometimes encountered in medical practice. The fact that they are connected is a total surprise. So are the tragic consequences of both diseases if they occur in one individual. The intractable pain and neurologic impairments are profound. The tears, depression, suffering, and suicide when the two diseases exist together is the underlying reason this book has been written. As unpleasant as it may be, there is no denying the EDS-AA connection. All concerned parties simply must accept that the connection is here and work to develop some strategies for prevention and care. This book is intended to jump-start the process.

INTRODUCTION

This book has primarily been written to inform all concerned parties that the combination of Ehlers-Danlos Syndrome (EDS) and adhesive arachnoiditis (AA) now exists in clinical practice. It is a tragic development. The two diseases in the same individual results in enormous misery, pain, and suffering. Untreated and uncontrolled, this dual disease combination eventually produces neurologic impairments, intractable pain, malnutrition, a bed-bound state, and premature death. Suicide is common. This book describes how the connection was discovered and how it can be recognized and treated. Although EDS is genetic and can't be prevented, AA is a complication of EDS and can be prevented. All people with EDS have to know they are at risk for AA and must take specific cautions and measures to prevent it.

1. DEFINITIONS OF EDS AND AA

Ehlers-Danlos Syndromes (EDS) are a group of inherited disorders caused by different genetic defects in collagen production or metabolism. [8,9,15,24,25,72] Collagen is a tough, fibrous, protein that is a building block essential to strengthen the connective tissue that holds tissues together while providing flexibility to the tissue. [15,23] The most common variation of EDS is called hypermobile EDS, and it is characterized by one's ability to overextend joints and skin. Some dozen or so less common variations of EDS have been identified and are now collectively called Hypermobile Spectrum Disorders. [48,72] In this book, unless otherwise stated, EDS only refers to the most common syndrome, hypermobile EDS.

The arachnoid membrane is the middle layer of the brain and spinal canal cover known as the meninges. Arachnoiditis was defined in the "Comprehensive Medical Dictionary" published by J. B. Lippincott Co. in 1873 as "inflammation of the arachnoid membrane."

Adhesive arachnoiditis (AA) in this book is a lower spinal canal inflammatory, nerve entrapment disease in which cauda equina nerves become attached to the arachnoid membrane by adhesions. [1,2] The cauda equina consists of about two dozen nerves (often called nerve roots) that hang down from the spinal cord. In this book AA refers only to the lumbar-sacral spinal canal, unless otherwise stated. The arachnoid membrane is the inner layer of the spinal canal covering in the lower section of the spine. The outer layer is called the dura. Cauda equina nerves at the sites of attachment to the arachnoid-dural cover form small, inflamed masses which entrap nerves that are connected to the feet, legs, bladder, intestine, sex organs, and skin below about the level of the umbilicus.

AA only develops when two conditions are present. First there must be inflammation in both cauda equina nerves and arachnoid membrane to form adhesions that glue the two together. Second, there must be an inflammatory process or generator that causes inflammation and adhesions to form in both the cauda equina nerves and arachnoid membrane.

2. HOW COMMOM IS THE EDS-AA CONNECTION?

EDS and AA both seem to be increasing in clinical practice. About a generation ago, these two diseases were rare and known to few medical practitioners. It is unclear whether the apparent increase is due to an actual rise in disease incidence or improved awareness and diagnosis. Both factors may be operative. Regardless it is now inappropriate to call either condition "rare" as has been the custom in the past.

The prevalence of EDS is generally accepted at about one in every 600 to 900 people. Recent studies suggest a prevalence of about 3 to 4% of the general population affecting 3.3% of women and .6% of men. [8,9,72] If the United States is considered to have a population of 330 million people, a 4% prevalence translates to about 15 million persons. Interestingly, some recent surveys suggest that today's children and teenagers may have a much higher prevalence than 4%. Why this is could be the case or whether the surveys are inaccurate is unknown.

I have previously published that AA is an old disease that has re-emerged in this century. Causation of the re-emergence is at least partially attributed to changes in lifestyle, health habits, and an increase in spinal medical procedures such as epidural injections and surgery. [13,20] The lifestyle and health habits that have caused an increase in intervertebral disc disorders include sedentary lifestyle, obesity, diets which promote diabetes, and lack of exercise. Intervertebral disc degeneration and protrusions almost always precede AA. Disc protrusions or herniations may produce spinal canal stenosis and chronic compression, friction, and inflammation of the cauda equina nerves which lead to AA.[1,39,67,73] Some reports have suggested that the advent of epidural corticosteroid injections have caused the rise in the incidence of AA[20].

The seeming increase in AA, at least in part, is also likely due to the advent of contrast magnetic resonance imaging (MRI) which can almost always identify AA.

In summary, both EDS and AA have emerged in recent years as diseases now observed in medical practice. Both diseases seem to be increasing both by an actual disease incidence as well as the ability to diagnose cases that previously went undetected.

3. HOW THE CONNECTION WAS DISCOVERED

A brief review on how the EDS-AA connection was discovered is described here both for historical and clinical purposes. The discovery highlights the point that every person with severe chronic back pain should be screened for both EDS and AA.

Beginning in the early part of this century, persons with EDS began to attend the authors intractable pain clinic. EDS is known to produce severe, chronic pain. [16,22,60,61,68,75]

Criteria to enter the author's clinic required the patient be referred due to failure of multiple medical treatments to relieve intractable pain. Patients were accepted if it was estimated they would likely reach terminus within one year without intractable pain care. Many patients at the time did not have a diagnosis of EDS or AA. These diagnoses came later. Maximal enrollment in the clinic was about 125 total patients of which the majority attended monthly or bi-monthly. This clinic was not for profit, and fees were below family practice standards or based on "ability-to-pay."

Between the mid-1970's and the end of the 20th century, the clinic treated intractable pain patients who primarily had metastatic cancer, post-viral or diabetic neuropathy, rheumatic diseases, reflex sympathetic dystrophy, sickle cell anemia, severe arthritis, or post head or spine trauma. In the latter part of the 20th and early 21st century, the spectrum of disease that caused intractable pain began to change. [13,41,53,69] New or better disease treatments had been developed. These treatments may not have been curative, but they prevented the development of intractable pain. Included in this category were specific treatments for rheumatic diseases, sickle cell anemia, arthritis, diabetes, and cancer. Patients with severe, disabling back pain emerged as the primary reason to seek intractable, pain care.

Almost all patients with intractable back pain had undergone surgical procedures and carried the medical diagnosis of "failed back surgery syndrome." [13] The surgery was almost always done for herniated discs, but it failed to relieve the patient's pain. "Failed back" wasn't a helpful diagnosis, so a concerted research effort was made to find the cause of "failure." Thanks to the technology and accuracy of magnetic resonance imaging (MRI), it soon became apparent that a high percentage of "failed back surgery" cases had AA.[1]

Initially our belief was that AA was a purely anatomic spine problem. This belief started to modify when a number of AA patients informed me that they had EDS. With this knowledge I began to inquire of all patients if they had EDS. We started to screen all patients with AA for the presence of EDS by use of the screening tools described in a later chapter. The results were somewhat astounding. At least 30 to 50% of patients with AA had EDS.

4. THE EHLERS-DANLOS SYNDROME (EDS)

EDS is an inherited or genetic disease in which the fundamental biologic defect is a deficit or deficiency of collagen. [8,15,28,57] Collagen deficiency may be quantitative or qualitative. The basic metabolic defect can be in either production or maintenance of collagen. In simple terms it is the "glue" that holds or connects tissues together. [23,57] For example, it attaches teeth to their socket. Of great relevance to the EDS-AA connection, adequate collagen is essential for maintenance of the arachnoid membrane which one of its functions is to hold together the spinal canal cover.

EDS is commonly called a "connective tissue disorder" because a defect in either quantity or quality of collagen causes tissues to be elastic and "stretchable." When one can stretch or extend their skin, joints, or extremities more than normal, such a person is termed "hypermobile." Hypermobility is due to collagen deficiency in ligaments, fascia, and other connective tissues that allows the joints to dislocate or overextend. A common description is "double-jointedness." A vivid example was the "rubber man" in the circus who could pull his neck and chest skin over his head.

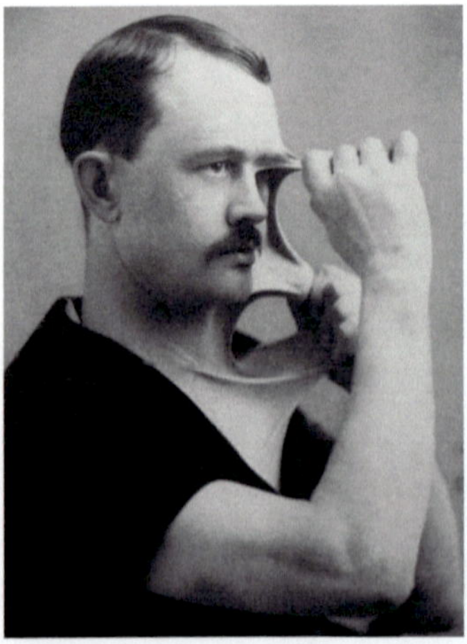 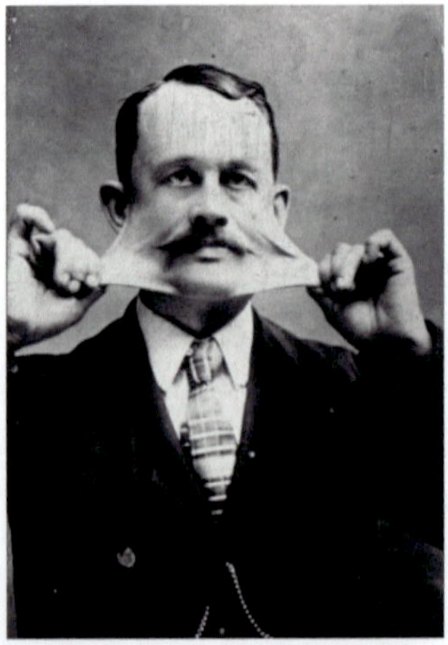

James Morris was known as "Rubberman" in the Barnum Circus of the last half of the 1800's. Morris had lax skin due to a genetic absence of collagen in his skin. This same absence of viable collagen may affect joints and internal organs such as the colon, eye, and spinal canal.

Patients with EDS often have skin that can be described as "velvety" or "loose." This skin characteristic predisposes patients to problems with wound healing. Patients will often note that they develop "paper-thin" scars. Fragile blood vessels may produce easy bruising, and bleeding gums can weaken teeth that may erode or fall out. Collagen defects may exist below the skin that obviously can't be visualized. Tissues such as blood vessels, blood cells, heart, intestines, spine and nerves may be defective.[7,17,63] Collagen deficiency may lead to tears, inflammation, degeneration, and scarring in connective tissues. Severe intractable pain and a variety of neurologic, immune, and metabolic complications may result. [7,10,31,46,60]

Normal collagen has other biologic roles besides holding tissues together. It protects tissues from tearing and resists infections and autoimmune degeneration (See figure). A major problem for persons with EDS is that collagen deficits make tissues vulnerable to trauma, infections, and autoimmune degeneration.

Doctors Ehlers and Danlos first described the disease. [17,19] In Paris in 1899, Dr. Lauritz Edvard Ehlers presented a law student with lax skin, a tendency to hematomas of the skin, and generalized loose joints to the French Dermatologic Society. In 1908, Dr. Henri Alexander Danlos presented to the French Dermatologic Society a boy with fragile and extensible skin. In honor of these two physicians the disease of "loose tissue" is called Ehlers-Danlos Syndrome.

After the discovery of EDS, it was pretty much considered, during the last century, a genetic oddity with few or no medical consequences. Its main notoriety was children who could "show off" to their friends their double joints, splits, and body contortions. Over-extension of joints and "hypermobility" were considered harmless and even revered, such as with the case of the famous singer, Elvis Presley, who could do amazing body extensions and contortions while performing on stage.

In the latter part of the last century, however, EDS began to be recognized as a genetic disease that may lead to severe medical complications. A clinical profile emerged, and a renowned geneticist, Dr. Peter Beighton, in 1997, developed the criteria for the diagnosis of EDS [4]. The most common form of EDS as noted previously in this book, is termed hypermobile EDS. About a dozen variations, however, have been described. The term hypermobile spectrum disorder is now the term applied to persons who have some skin or joint laxity and other evidence of collagen deficiency but don't meet the Beighton profile. The Beighton diagnostic criteria remains the standard diagnostic tool for EDS as no blood or genetic test has yet been developed. The Beighton criteria and scoring system is in Chapter Seven.

EDS causes a wide variety of symptoms and complications. The attached Table provides a quick summary of the common complications of EDS. Although EDS is primarily thought to be a disease of skin and joints, it is associated with multiple mental and metabolic abnormalities that may destabilize the autonomic (involuntary) nervous system and cause such symptoms as tachycardia, syncope, dizziness, brain fog, anxiety, sleep deprivation, and dysregulated temperature and blood pressure control (dysautonomia).[7,10,15,28,72]

EDS has significant immune deficiency. Mast cells may over activate to produce symptoms such as flushing, hives, fatigue, anaphylaxis, and malaise. Unfortunately, EDS immune deficiency makes the individual prone to develop infections. Bacteria, such as Lyme and mycobacteria, commonly affect persons with EDS. Virus infections are extremely problematic. The Epstein-Barr Virus (EBV) has emerged as a causative factor in several diseases as noted later in this book. It seems to have a predilection for persons with EDS. This normal parasitic virus may reactivate and produce an autoimmune state that can lead to several pathologic complications including multiple sclerosis, some cancers, rheumatic diseases, and AA.

Intractable, severe pain defined as constant pain with cardiovascular, endocrine (hormone), immunologic, and metabolic complications is extremely problematic in EDS.[16,68,75] Small fiber neuropathy is essentially universal in EDS, and it may cause severe pain "all over." [36] Joints, muscles, and fascia may be affected and cause pain. Neural problems including AA are detailed in later chapters. When combined with AA, intractable pain may require the most aggressive pain relief drugs including opioids, amphetamine derivatives, and benzodiazepines. Implanted electrical modulators and opioid infusion devices may be required for adequate pain control.

A number of excellent clinicians have recently published their symptomatic or ameliorative treatments for the main complications of EDS. These treatments have been well-catalogued in two recent books that are highly recommended to medical practitioners: (1) "Symptomatic" edited by Clair Francomano, et al; and (2) "Disjointed" edited by D. Jovin.

No specific treatment has emerged for EDS. This author highly recommends therapies and measures directed at collagen and tissue regeneration. These measures are primarily peptides and hormones that have anabolic or regenerative properties. [14,42,58] Although there are no systematic, reported studies by this author or any other, I believe we are seeing some positive, clinical improvement in pain and symptom relief with the combined use of some peptides and anabolic hormones. Some specifics are given in the later chapter on treatment.

TABLE
SOME COMMON MEDICAL COMPLICATIONS OF EDS

- Intractable pain
- Joint instability and hyper-extension, sprains, strains, subluxations, and/or dislocations
- Stomach and digestive problems (like reflux and slow stomach emptying)
- Poor proprioception (balance)
- Bladder and bowel problems
- Autonomic dysfunction including postural tachycardia syndrome (e.g. dizziness, fainting, light-headedness, difficulty regulating temperature)
- Easy bruising
- Poor wound healing
- Long term (persistent) pain
- Stretchy or soft skin
- Chronic fatigue
- Arthritis
- Small fiber neuropathy
- Neuropathies: pudendal, feet, face, mouth
- Spinal cord/canal inflammation disorders (e.g., leaks, Tarlov cysts, herniated discs, adhesive arachnoiditis, chronic cauda equina inflammation)

5. THE EDS ATTACK ON SPINE AND NEURAL TISSUES

EDS has multiple, serious neurologic complications.[10,11,12,21,26,31,36,47,56,64,65,66] The arachnoid membrane is the inner layer of the spinal canal cover. It is composed of fine neural tissue with high levels of collagen. It was so named because it looks like a spider web if viewed under a microscope. The outer layer, the dura, is thicker and tougher, and also contains a high level of collagen. Due to the collagen defect of EDS the spinal canal cover may be seriously affected. First, if the arachnoid layer weakens, a "bubble" or cyst known as a Tarlov cyst may develop inside the spinal canal. Second, tears or splits to the collagen matrix of the spinal canal cover may cause a spinal fluid leak. Some persons develop a spinal fluid leak before they are even aware they have EDS.[63] Third, chronic inflammation may develop in the arachnoid membrane. This condition, simply known as arachnoiditis, may spread inflammation to cauda equina nerves and set the stage for AA.[5]

EDS is now clearly known to cause small fiber neuropathy throughout the body. [11,21,36] Small nerve fibers are connected to a main nerve below the skin. They are anatomically connected between the skin surface and a main nerve. The purpose of the small fibers is to transmit the body's natural electricity production to the skin and into the air. If small nerve fibers are dysfunctional or eliminated, electricity and possibly some toxic substances may be retained just under the skin. This result is severe, burning pain. Major anatomic areas for small fiber neuropathy and burning pain are the feet, mouth, and perineal/groin areas. Persons with AA are especially prone to groin-crotch burning, pain since the major nerve that innervates the area is the pudendal nerve that emanates from cauda equina nerves that are entrapped and inflamed in AA. This condition is now commonly called pudendal neuropathy or neuralgia. Small fiber neuropathy is essentially universal in persons with EDS. It is probably the major cause of intractable pain in most persons with EDS. The apparent explanation is that small nerve fibers are thin and loaded with collagen that degenerate over time. It is unclear if the degeneration is principally caused by genetic programming or caused by autoimmunity. It is also unclear if the generator of autoimmunity is purely EDS or if it is Epstein-Barr Virus or other parasitic autoimmunity. Small fiber neuropathies have proven, until this time, to be resistant to a multitude of treatments. [26,34,52,65,70]

Cauda equina nerves, at least in some persons with EDS, appear to be part of the "small fiber neuropathy complication." Cauda equina nerves are thin, flexible, and literally dangling in spinal fluid when one stands. It may be that cauda equina nerves become inflamed and degenerate in tandem with small fiber neuropathy outside the spinal canal since they are both fine, small nerves with a high collagen content.

In order for a person with EDS to develop AA, inflammation must occur in both cauda equina nerves and arachnoid membrane. Inflammation in both tissues eventually forms adhesions that glue the two together. EDS has multiple characteristics that render a person with this condition to be at high risk for AA. Collagen deficiency followed by inflammation and adhesions may initially occur in either or both neural tissues. Autoimmune attack and degeneration may be due to EDS, per se, or be facilitated by EBV or other form of autoimmunity. [3,30,49,76]

Autoimmunity is simply defined here as a disease process or element in the body that attacks and destroys its own tissue. It is clear that EDS is highly associated with autoimmunity that attacks neural tissues. At this time, it is unclear whether EDS forms its own, innate autoimmunity or if it is caused by parasitic autoimmunity or other possible process. It is also possible that multiple types of autoimmunity may co-exist.

TABLE

EDS AFFECTS ON SPINAL CANAL COVER

- Tarlov cysts
- Spinal fluid leaks
- Non-adhesive arachnoiditis

FIGURE
COLLAGEN DEFICIENCY IN TISSUES

Normal collagen is in thick strands that hold tissues together and resist infections, tearing, and autoimmune degeneration.

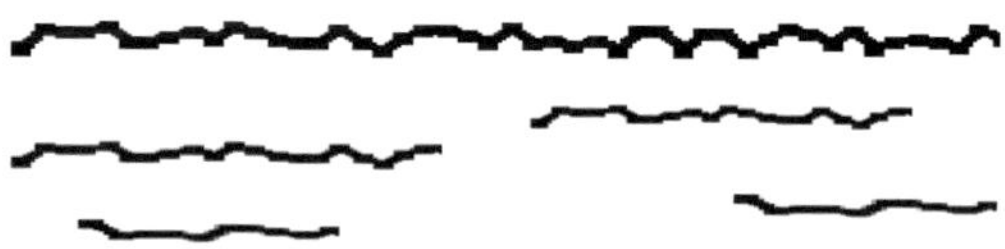

Deficient collagen strands may be thin, broken, shortened, or non-existent. Deficient collagen may tear and allow infections and autoimmune degeneration.

FIGURE
SMALL FIBER NEUROPATHY

Normal Small Fiber Neuropathy

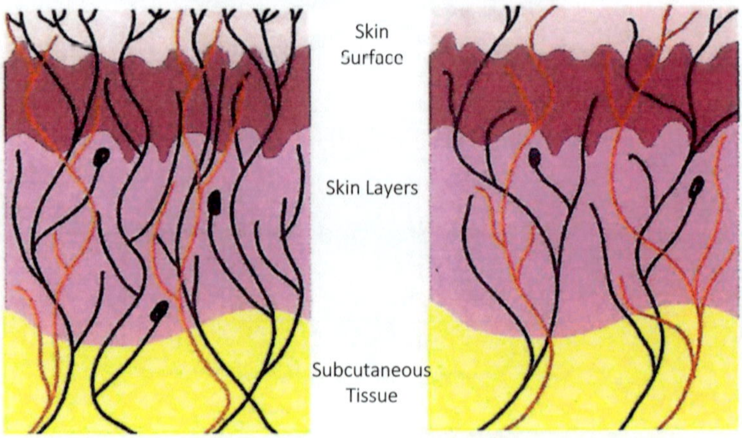

The picture on the left is normal skin showing a large number of small nerve fibers. The picture on the right shows a smaller number of nerve fibers. Neuropathy in this case means "lack or loss of fibers." The loss of small nerve fibers prohibits the normal conduction of bioelectricity which results in burning pain. This condition, if widespread, causes pain "all over."

6. RECOGNITION OF EDS

This book is primarily focused on the identification of the most common Ehlers-Danlos syndrome (EDS) which is now called hypermobile. Throughout this book only the common hypermobile EDS is emphasized, although there are about a dozen uncommon variations of EDS now collectively called Hypermobile Spectrum Disorder.

Described here are simple screening tests and risk factors to help identify the person with EDS. In the past, many cases of EDS weren't diagnosed until the person who had it reached middle age. Simply put, this book is focused on assisting persons with EDS to be diagnosed in childhood or young adulthood so hopefully the connection of EDS-AA can be either prevented or ameliorated.

The following Table points out some clinical manifestations and risk factors that call for EDS screening.

TABLE

Risk Factors that Warrant Screening for EDS

- Persons with intractable pain
- Growing pains as a child
- History of problem pregnancy
- History of infectious mononucleosis, Tarlov cyst, spinal fluid leak
- Failed back surgery
- Severe back pain for over 90 days

Two screening tests for EDS have been promulgated in recent years. They are simple and can quickly be administered in any clinical setting or through email or mail.

The first screen is a simple five-question instrument developed by the well-known EDS experts, Drs. A.J. Hakim and R. Grahame in London, England. [27]

TABLE

Five Question Screen for EDS

1. Do you consider yourself double-jointed? Yes/No
2. Can you now or could you ever place your hands flat on the floor without bending your knees? Yes/No
3. Can you now or could you ever bend your thumb back to your forearm? Yes/No
4. As a child, did you amuse your friends by contorting your body into strange shapes or could you do the splits? Yes/No
5. As a child or teenager, did your shoulder or kneecap dislocate on more than one occasion? Yes/No

A yes answer to two questions suggests you have an 80% probability of having EDS.

Reference: Hakim AJ, Grahame R. A simple questionnaire to detect hypermobility: an adjunct to the assessment of patients with diffuse musculoskeletal pain. *Int J Clin Pract* 2003;57:163-166.

In 2017, Drs. C. Hamonet and L Ducret developed a twelve-question screen [28]. If you answered yes to five or more of the twelve screening questions, the doctors found that you have about a 98% chance you have EDS.

TABLE

	TWELVE QUESTION SCREEN FOR EDS	**Yes**	**No**
1	Do you have pain in multiple locations?		
2	Do you have extreme fatigue?		
3	Are you clumsy sometimes and fall or walk into objects?		
4	Are some of the joints in your hands, feet, elbow, hips or knees “loose” or quite flexible?		
5	Have you had a lot of sprains or joint dislocations?		
6	Is your skin thin in places?		
7	Are you double-jointed or able to bend your fingers, arms, or ankle backward?		
8	Are your hands and feet cold much of the time?		
9	Do you bruise easily or have bruises that suddenly occur?		
10	Is your skin “stretchy” in some places?		
11	Are you constipated a lot?		
12	Do you suffer from “heart burn” or frequent episodes of food regurgitation?		
Hamonet C, Ducret L. Ehlers-Danlos, an unknown and disturbing syndrome, free comments. *Theranostics Brain, Spine, and Neurol Disord* 2017;2:555-591.			

If a person has a positive response to either of the above screening tests, EDS is confirmed with a Beighton Score. The committed and energetic, Ehlers-Danlos Society provides a standard Beighton criteria and score form for any medical practitioner. I have placed a Beighton Diagnostic Score form in this chapter.

The author has developed a supplementary set of questions to help diagnose collagen deficiency diseases other than hypermobile EDS. This questionnaire is in the Appendix. Its use is to help diagnose an unusual EDS variant (Hypermobile Spectrum Disorder) or a connective tissue, collagen deficiency disease such as Marfan syndrome.

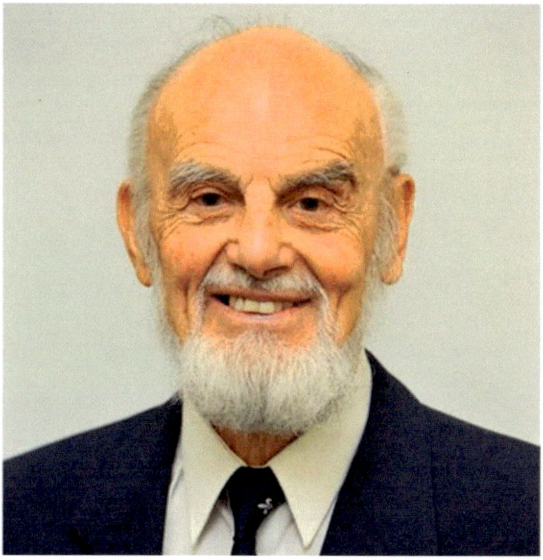

In 1997, renowned geneticist, Dr. Peter Beighton developed the criteria for the clinical diagnosis of EDS. His diagnostic scoring system is on the next page.

Diagnostic Criteria for Hypermobile Ehlers-Danlos Syndrome (hEDS)

CRITERION 1 – Generalized Joint Hypermobility

One of the following selected:

- ☐ ≥6 pre-pubertal children and adolescents
- ☐ ≥5 pubertal men and woman to age 50
- ☐ ≥4 men and women over the age of 50

Beighton Score: ____/9

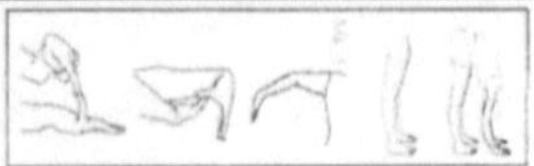

If Beighton Score is one point below age- and sex-specific cut off, two or more of the following must also be selected to meet criterion:

- ☐ Can you now (or could you ever) place your hands flat on the floor without bending your knees?
- ☐ Can you now (or could you ever) bend your thumb to touch your forearm?
- ☐ As a child, did you amuse your friends by contorting your body into strange shapes or could you do the splits?
- ☐ As a child or teenager, did your shoulder or kneecap dislocate on more than one occasion?
- ☐ Do you consider yourself "double jointed"?

CRITERION 2 – Two or more of the following features (A, B, or C) must be present

Feature A (five must be present)

- ☐ Unusually soft or velvety skin
- ☐ Mild skin hyperextensibility
- ☐ Unexplained striae distensae or rubae at the back, groins, thighs, breasts and/or abdomen in adolescents, men or pre-pubertal women without a history of significant gain or loss of body fat or weight
- ☐ Bilateral piezogenic papules of the heel
- ☐ Recurrent or multiple abdominal hernia(s)
- ☐ Atrophic scarring involving at least two sites and without the formation of truly papyraceous and/or hemosideric scars as seen in classical EDS
- ☐ Pelvic floor, rectal, and/or uterine prolapse in children, men or nulliparous women without a history of morbid obesity or other known predisposing medical condition
- ☐ Dental crowding and high or narrow palate
- ☐ Arachnodactyly, as defined in one or more of the following:
  (i) positive wrist sign (Walker sign) on both sides, (ii) positive thumb sign (Steinberg sign) on both sides
- ☐ Arm span-to-height ratio ≥1.05
- ☐ Mitral valve prolapse (MVP) mild or greater based on strict echocardiographic criteria
- ☐ Aortic root dilatation with Z-score >+2

Feature A total: ____/12

Feature B

- ☐ Positive family history; one or more first-degree relatives independently meeting the current criteria for hEDS

Feature C (must have at least one)

- ☐ Musculoskeletal pain in two or more limbs, recurring daily for at least 3 months
- ☐ Chronic, widespread pain for ≥3 months
- ☐ Recurrent joint dislocations or frank joint instability, in the absence of trauma

CRITERION 3 - All of the following prerequisites MUST be met

1. Absence of unusual skin fragility, which should prompt consideration of other types of EDS
2. Exclusion of other heritable and acquired connective tissue disorders, including autoimmune rheumatologic conditions. In patients with an acquired CTD (e.g. Lupus, Rheumatoid Arthritis, etc.), additional diagnosis of hEDS requires meeting both Features A and B of Criterion 2. Feature C of Criterion 2 (chronic pain and/or instability) cannot be counted toward a diagnosis of hEDS in this situation.
3. Exclusion of alternative diagnoses that may also include joint hypermobility by means of hypotonia and/or connective tissue laxity. Alternative diagnoses and diagnostic categories include, but are not limited to, neuromuscular disorders (e.g. Bethlem myopathy), other hereditary disorders of the connective tissue (e.g. other types of EDS, Loeys-Dietz syndrome, Marfan syndrome), and skeletal dysplasias (e.g. osteogenesis imperfecta). Exclusion of these considerations may be based upon history, physical examination, and/or molecular genetic testing, as indicated.

This form is graciously supplied as a public service to any medical practitioner by the "Ehlers-Danlos Society" and the "International Consortium of Ehlers-Danlos Syndromes and Related Disorders."

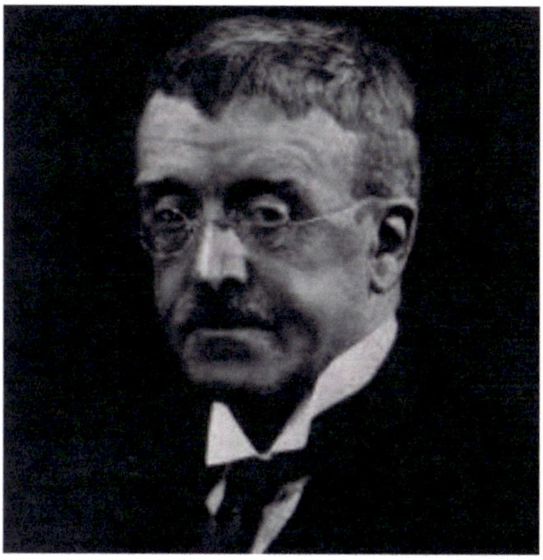

In 1899, Dr. Edvard Lauritz Ehlers presented the first case, a law student with lax skin and joints, to the French Dermatologic Society in Paris, France.

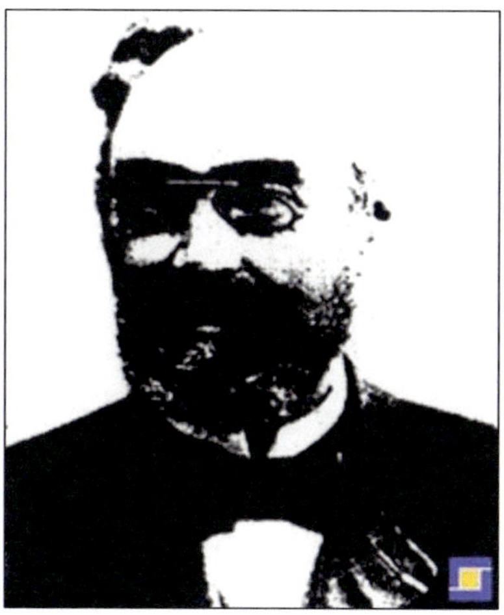

In 1908, Dr. Henri Danlos presented to the French Dermatologic Society a second case, a boy with fragile and extensible skin.

7. ADHESIVE ARACHNOIDITIS: THE DEVIL'S DISEASE

AA is an inflammatory nerve entrapment disease of the lumbar-sacral spine in which cauda equina nerves become adhered (glued) by adhesions to the inner lining (arachnoid membrane) of the spinal canal cover (meninges).[1,2,5] At the site where cauda equina nerves and arachnoid membrane are attached, a mass (clump) is formed that entraps nerves, blocks spinal fluid flow, and will usually erode through the canal covering and leak spinal fluid into non-spinal tissues. [37,71] Unless appropriately treated, intractable pain, multiple neurologic impairments, and premature death will occur. [59] Suicide is common in undertreated persons.

AA was often referred to as a "devil's disease" in the 1800's. No wonder. It' pathologic complications of intractable pain, malnutrition, paralysis, dementia, and early death rightfully invoked dread and sorrow for patients and families. Two of Dr. Thomas Addison's eleven adrenal failure cases, which he reported in 1855, had anatomic evidence of AA in the lumbar-sacral spine. In 1873 arachnoiditis was defined in the Comprehensive Medical Dictionary as an "inflammatory disease of the arachnoid membrane."

In the 1800's and early 1900's AA was usually caused by tuberculosis or syphilis. Due to the advent of antibiotics in the mid-1900's, AA essentially disappeared and was classified as a rare disease. Essentially, the only known cases in the latter part of the last century were those that occasionally occurred as a complication of dyes used for myelograms. With the invention of magnetic resonance imaging (MRI) in the late 1980's, toxic dyes were seldom used in myelograms. Consequently, AA almost became a forgotten disease. Exactly why AA has re-emerged as a disease in this century is somewhat unclear. The ability to diagnose it by a typical clinical profile and MRI have certainly contributed to its increased recognition. Herniated intervertebral discs almost always precede AA, so factors that promote disc degeneration such as obesity, sedentary lifestyle, and smoking may be causative factors. Surgery and epidural injections for disc disease may contribute to AA's apparent increase. Autoimmunity is increasing in incidence for multiple reasons and autoimmunity can affect spinal canal tissues.

AA only develops when two conditions are present. First, inflammation in both cauda equina nerves and arachnoid membrane must exist in order that adhesions can form and glue the two tissues together. Second, there must be one or more generators or initiators of inflammation in the spinal canal tissues. These include autoimmune disorder, trauma, infections, and the presence of a toxic substance in spinal fluid. As often as not, the person with AA may have multiple generators of inflammation. The Table here lists the usual generators of spinal canal inflammation. [5] A collagen deficiency disease, especially EDS, enables inflammation to be more easily generated in spinal canal tissues.

Inflammation in cauda equina nerves and arachnoid membrane are almost always preceded by inflammation in intervertebral discs, ligamentum flavum (support ligament of the spine), and vertebrae. [18,39,55,67,73]

The severity of AA is classified into four categories or stages: (1) mild, (2) moderate, (3) severe, (4) catastrophic. A Table of categories and stages is in the Appendix. It is noted that symptom relief and clinical improvement respond best in mild and moderate cases. Persons in the severe category generally do less well. The catastrophic stage requires palliative measures.

TABLE
GENERATORS OF SPINAL CANAL INFLAMMATION

1. Autoimmune disorder from a rheumatic disease or parasitic virus such as Epstein-Barr
2. Toxic substance in spinal fluid introduced by a canal opening or puncture
3. Friction or compression of cauda equina nerves from an anatomic abnormality usually scoliosis, spinal stenosis, or ankylosing spondylitis
4. Trauma from accident or medical procedure
5. Infectious agent usually Lyme or Epstein-Barr Virus

Note: The presence of a collagen deficiency disease such as EDS makes spinal canal tissues more susceptible to the development of inflammation.

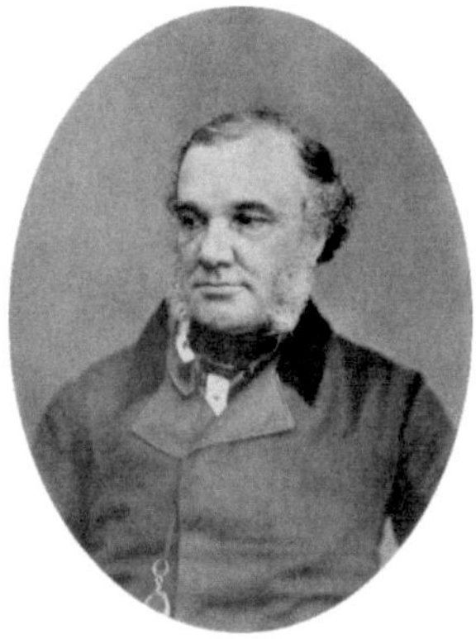

Dr. Thomas Addison in 1855 published a monograph on his discovery of adrenal failure and its clinical manifestations. Two of his eleven cases showed evidence of adhesive arachnoiditis.

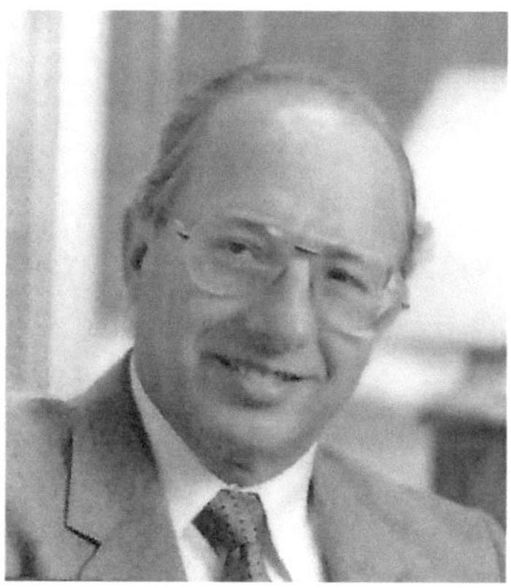

Dr. Jorge Antonio Aldrete pioneered emergency treatment for AA, developed MRI analysis for AA, and determined that a high percentage of persons called "failed back syndrome" have AA. He was the personal mentor on AA for the author.

LEAKAGE DIAGRAM

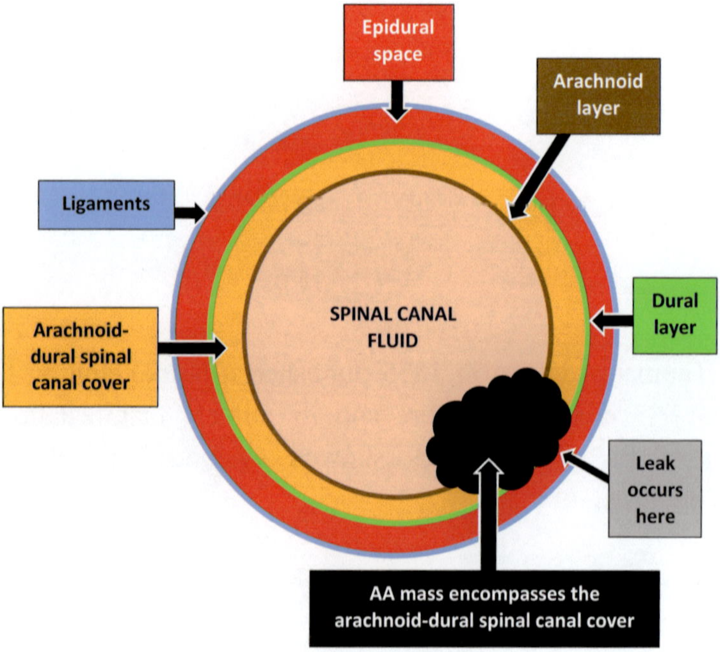

Almost all cases of AA will develop seepage or leakage of spinal fluid at the site where cauda equina nerves become attached to the spinal canal cover.

Diagram of Entrapped Nerve Roots in AA

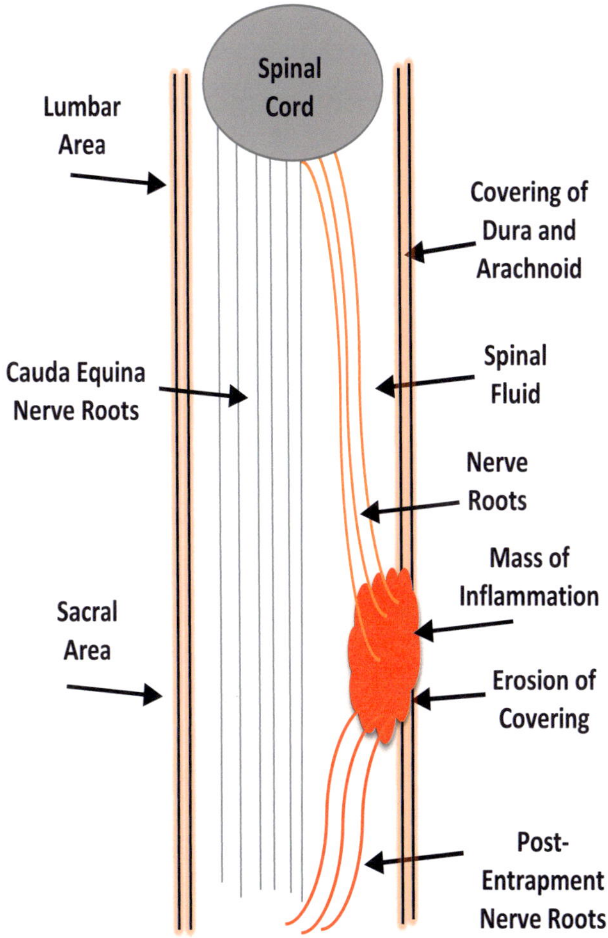

Depending on which cauda equina nerves are entrapped will determine specific clinical symptoms. Most AA nerve entrapments affect the bladder, bowel, legs, and feet.

8. PATHOLOGIC COMPLICATIONS OF AA

AA has four major classes of pathologic complications. The disease may be progressive with exacerbations and remissions, so complications may come in steps or stages. Severe intractable pain is usually the most devastating symptom for persons with the disease. Suicide has been common with undertreated AA but, based on personal observations and reports, it seems to be decreasing with recognition and treatment. Intractable pain is actually a syndrome which causes multiple endocrine, cardiovascular, immune, and metabolic abnormalities. Among the endocrine complications is adrenal exhaustion and even failure. In the 1800's adrenal failure was probably the most common cause of death in persons with AA. Today, the cause of death in AA may include systemic infections or cardiac arrest.

The major pathologic complications are related to inflammation, cauda equina nerve entrapment, and spinal fluid flow impairment or leakage. Inflammation in cauda equina nerves causes pain and other symptoms such as the sensation of water dripping or insects crawling on the skin. Entrapment of nerves leads to burning feet, and neurologic impairments of bladder, intestine, sex organs, legs, and feet. The inflamed adhesive mass inside the spinal canal blocks spinal fluid flow and may erode through the arachnoid-dura covering of the spinal canal and permit spinal fluid to leak into the tissues that surrounds the spine. [32]

The attached Table summarizes many of the pathologic complications of AA. A glance at the Table provides ample reason for an aggressive approach to early recognition and prevention of the disease.

TABLE
PATHOLOGIC COMPLICATIONS OF AA

PATHOLOGIC DEVELOPMENT	SOME COMPLICATIONS
Inflammation with Nerve Destruction	Intractable pain with hormone suppression, hypertension, tachycardia, adrenal failure, cardiac arrest, premature death, burning pains in feet and perineal area
Entrapment of Cauda Equina Nerves	Leg/ankle/foot paralysis, bladder impairment (hesitancy, frequency, incontinence), bowel impairment (bloating, pain, alternating constipation and diarrhea), pain when sitting, sex organ paralysis (penis, vagina), weakness, loss of balance, falls
Spinal Fluid Flow Obstruction/Alteration	Headache, blurred vision, tinnitus (ringing in ears), nasal dripping, vertigo
Spinal Fluid Leakage into Back Tissues	Skin indentation, muscles contract, arm/neck extension reduced, back pain

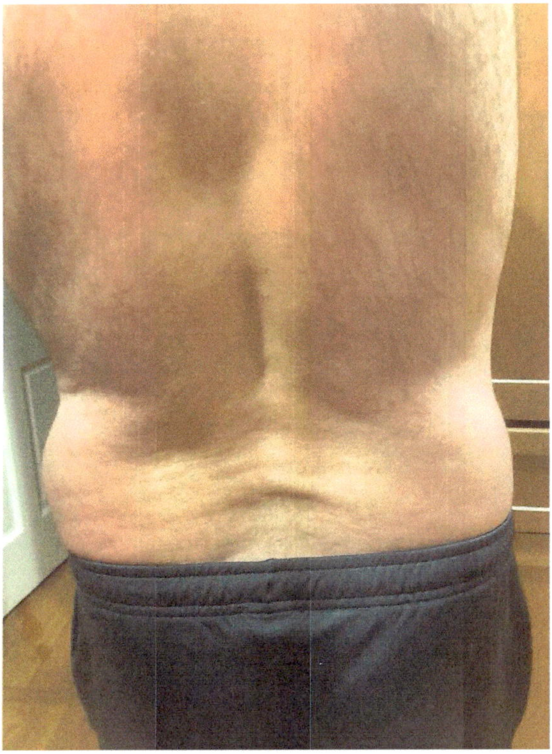

This person with AA and EDS has not had surgery. Note midline indentation and skin-muscle contractures. He splints to the left as indicated by a skin crease. Medical practitioners should suspect AA if a patient presents with multiple anatomical abnormalities and asymmetry of the lower back.

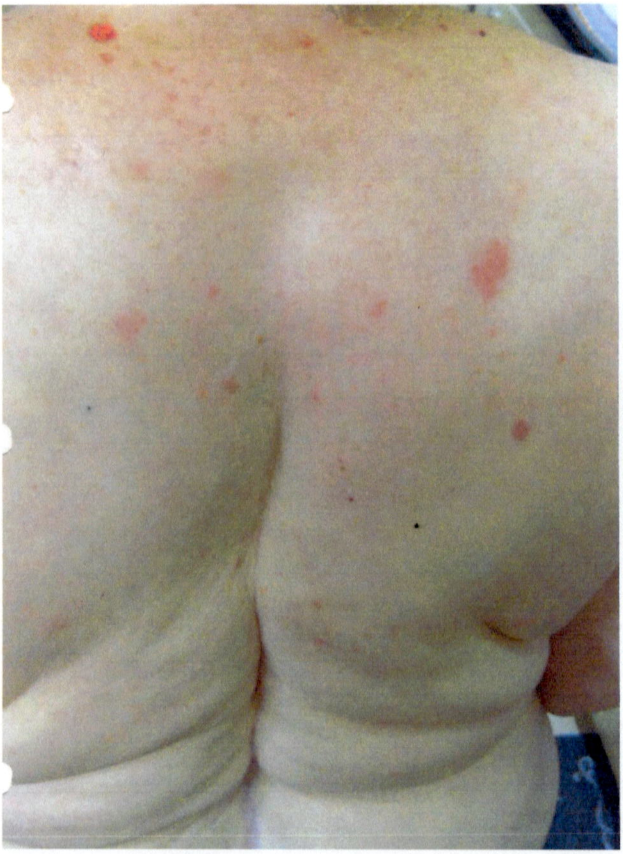

Note: There is distortion of muscle structure, skin contractures, and midline indentations. Patient is post-surgical (laminectomy). AA was confirmed in this patient with EDS by contrast MRI of the lumbar-sacral spine.

Back of AA Patient

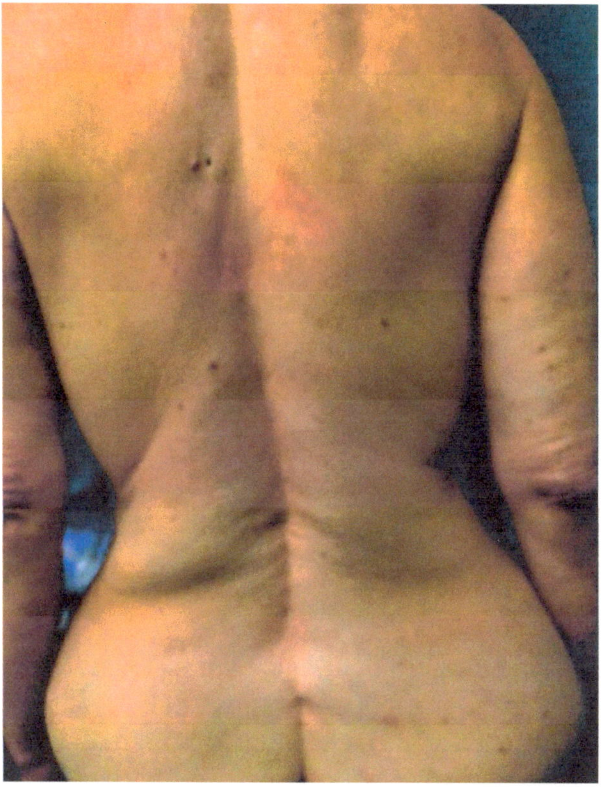

Note distorted muscle structure, skin contractures, asymmetry, and midline indentations. Patient is post-surgical (lumbar fusion). She splints to the left as indicated by a skin crease. EDS and AA progress over a considerable time period that is reflected by multiple anatomic abnormalities of the back.

9. PERSONS WITH EDS AT HIGH RISK OF AA

AA is the end result or culmination of multiple pathologic stages and biologic events. It does not occur until there is inflammation in both cauda equina nerves and the inner lining of the spinal canal cover (arachnoid membrane). If inflammation is in both tissues, adhesions may form which adhere or "glue" the two tissues together. AA is always preceded and accompanied by other spinal canal inflammatory disorders and conditions. MRI analysis of AA cases routinely shows evidence of inflammation in multiple spine tissue including discs, vertebrae, ligamentum flavum, and filum terminal. [18,73]

There are four spinal inflammatory conditions which are commonly present in a person with EDS before AA develops. In fact, any of the four spinal conditions listed in the Table may be the first indication in a person with EDS that they have serious spine complications. (See Table below) If a person with EDS has one of the four conditions in the Table, they need to aggressively take measures to prevent AA.

TABLE
FOUR SPINAL INFLAMMATORY CONDITIONS THAT MAY PRECEDE AA

Herniated discs	Tarlov cyst
Spinal Canal Leak	Tethered cord

In many cases of the combined diseases of EDS and AA, the person will have herniated discs in both the cervical and lumbar-sacral regions of the spine. It is also noted that persons with EDS who have spinal taps or epidural corticoid injections are prone to develop pain, sciatica, and delirium after the procedure. They often go on to develop AA. If a person with EDS develops spine pain and an inflammatory spinal condition, an aggressive effort must be made to determine the precise causes of the inflammation and suppress it to prevent the development of AA.

10. WHO TO SUSPECT AND EVALUATE FOR AA

Recognition and clinical diagnosis of AA is only possible when it is suspected. It should be recognized, diagnosed, and treated as early as possible. Those persons with AA in the mild and moderate stages fare much better in treatment than those persons in stages three (severe) and four (catastrophic). Back pain is usually a common, temporary symptom. AA is neither common nor temporary. It is the person with severe back pain that "hasn't gone away" after about 90 days despite treatment attempts. The major reason to suspect AA is, therefore, the person with back pain that doesn't go away if standard and usual medical measures haven't removed the pain. For example, most people will try to treat their back pain with heat, anti-inflammatories, chiropractic measures, or physical therapy when it first occurs. If these standard and usual treatments don't work, suspect AA. One of the major reasons to screen for AA are persons labeled with "failed back surgery syndrome." [1,13]

TABLE
PERSONS TO SCREEN FOR AA

- ✓ Back pain for over 90 days that requires daily medication
- ✓ Two or more back surgeries
- ✓ Diagnosis of "failed back surgery syndrome"
- ✓ Spine injury
- ✓ Anatomic, structural spine abnormality such as scoliosis or spinal stenosis
- ✓ Ankylosing spondylitis or psoriatic arthritis
- ✓ Lyme disease
- ✓ EDS

We have developed a screening test for AA. If one answers yes to four of the seven questions, AA is very likely present. Confirmation of AA is done with a physical examination, history, and contrast lumbar-sacral MRI.

	SCREENING, DIAGNOSTIC TEST FOR AA	Yes	No
1	In addition to chronic pain, do you ever experience sharp, stabbing pains in your lower back or buttocks when you twist, turn or bend?		
2	Do you experience bizarre skin sensations such as crawling insects or water dripping down one or both legs?		
3	Do you experience burning pains in your feet and/or groin/crotch area?		
4	Does your pain lessen for a while when you stand or recline?		
5	Do you have leg or foot weakness and sometimes lose your balance and fall?		
6	Do you experience any bladder dysfunction such as dribbling, or difficulty when starting or stopping urination?		
7	Do you sometimes have blurred vision?		
If four or more questions are answered "yes" and the person taking the test has had constant back pain over 90 days, the person should be further evaluated for the presence of AA.			

Special Note: Chronic cauda equina inflammation may cause all the symptoms referred to in the above screening test. If AA is not observed on MRI, the person may appropriately be labeled "Cauda Equina Inflammatory Disorder."

11. DIAGNOSIS OF AA

AA, like other chronic diseases, is diagnosed by a systematic process. In the case of AA, the diagnosis is made by a typical history, symptom profile, physical abnormalities, and confirmed by a lumbar-sacral MRI.

<u>History</u>

1. Back pain over 90 days that has not resolved with standard physical and medical measures.

2. Presence of a causative or risk factor.
   - a. Structural, anatomic spine defect (scoliosis, spondylolisthesis, spinal stenosis)
   - b. Heritable connective tissue disorder (Ehlers-Danlos, Marfan Syndrome)
   - c. Autoimmune disorder (ankylosing spondylitis, systemic lupus, rheumatoid arthritis, psoriasis, parasitic viral, especially Epstein-Barr)
   - d. Trauma to brain or spine (accident, medical procedure)
   - e. Brain/spine infection (Lyme or virus)

Common Symptoms

1. Back and buttock pain that radiates to legs
2. Bladder dysfunction (hesitancy, dripping, can't stop)
3. Bizarre skin sensation (crawling insects, water dripping)
4. Burning feet and/or perineal area
5. Leg and/or foot weakness
6. Positional pain (temporarily improved by standing/sitting)
7. Blurred vision
8. Uncontrolled diarrhea

Common Physical Abnormalities

1. Leg weakness - one side is common
2. Pain on straight leg raising or rotation of hips
3. Loss touch/vibration sensation in foot, ankles, cold to the touch
4. Restriction of range of motion in arms and/or legs
5. Decreased reflexes - unilateral
6. Pain on pressure over lower lumbar-sacral area
7. Asymmetry and distortion of back musculature
8. Indentation of mid-back/spine area

Laboratory Tests for Excess Inflammation

1. Erythrocyte sedimentation rate (ESR)
2. C-reactive protein (CRP)
3. White blood cell count
4. Leukotrienes/cytokines

Confirmation

Final confirmation of AA is done with a contrast magnetic resonance imaging (MRI) study of the lumbar-sacral spinal canal. Contrast refers to the ability to differentiate spinal fluid from solid tissues. Two basic MRI views are used: (1) axial (toe to head) so the inside of the canal and cauda equina nerves can be visualized and analyzed; (2) a side or lateral (sagittal) view.

TABLE
Common MRI findings of AA

AXIAL IMAGES (Toe to Head) OF CAUDA EQUINA NERVES	**SAGITTAL IMAGES (Lateral View) OF SPINE AND CANAL**
√ Enlarged √ Displaced √ Clumped/coalesced √ Adherence of nerves to spinal canal covering (peripheralization) √ Asymmetry √ Lack of space between nerves	√ Dilated canal (empty sac) √ Nerves enlarged √ Spinal fluid outside canal √ Non-filling defects √ Protruding discs/stenosis

An MRI diagnosis of AA is made when a group of cauda equina nerves have coalesced or clumped into a small mass that is adhered or glued to the inner lining (arachnoid) of the spinal canal cover. The Table here describes the finding of cauda equina nerves which suggest the presence of inflammation and adhesions. Inflamed cauda equina nerves will usually show enlargement due to inflammation and edema. The nerves will usually be displaced from their normal symmetrical pattern. Some nerves may stick together and show little spacing between them. If clumping and adherence of cauda equina nerves to the arachnoid membrane are not observed but nerves show evidence of inflammation, it may be appropriate to use the label "cauda equina inflammatory disorder."

MRI of Person with EDS

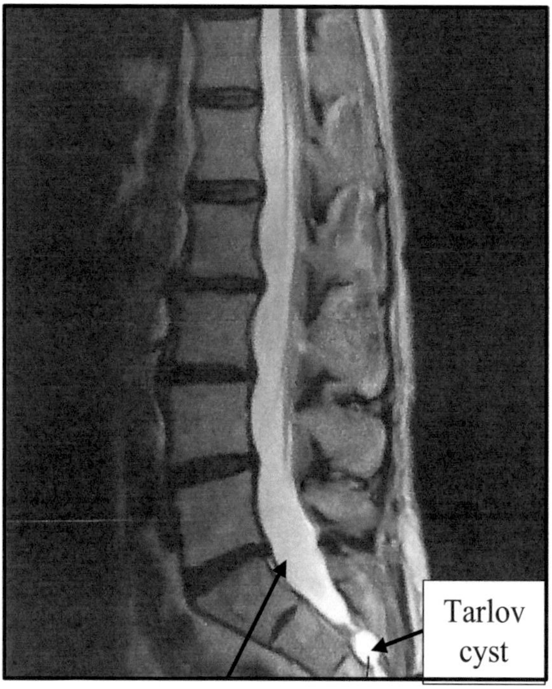

Dilated or "empty sac." Multiple discs press upon the spinal canal. A cyst is in the spinal canal. This patient must walk with a walker, has intermittent gastroparesis, severe constipation, and incontinence. Pain is severe, constant, and requires opioid suppression. This person has EDS and collagen deficiency which may result in a dilated canal and Tarlov cyst.

MRI: Spinal Fluid Leakage in AA

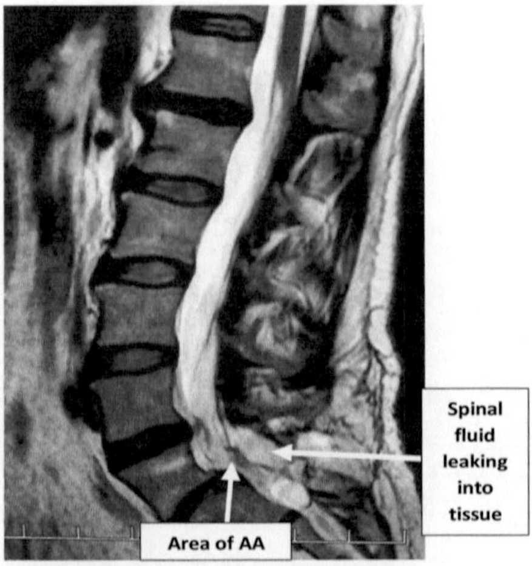

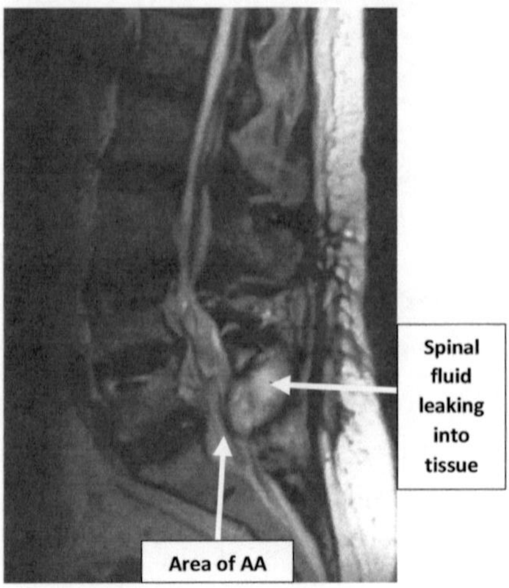

MRI images showing spinal fluid leaks around the area of AA. Person with EDS are prone to leaks due to a collagen deficient, "weakened" spinal canal cover.

MRI: Catastrophic Case of AA and EDS

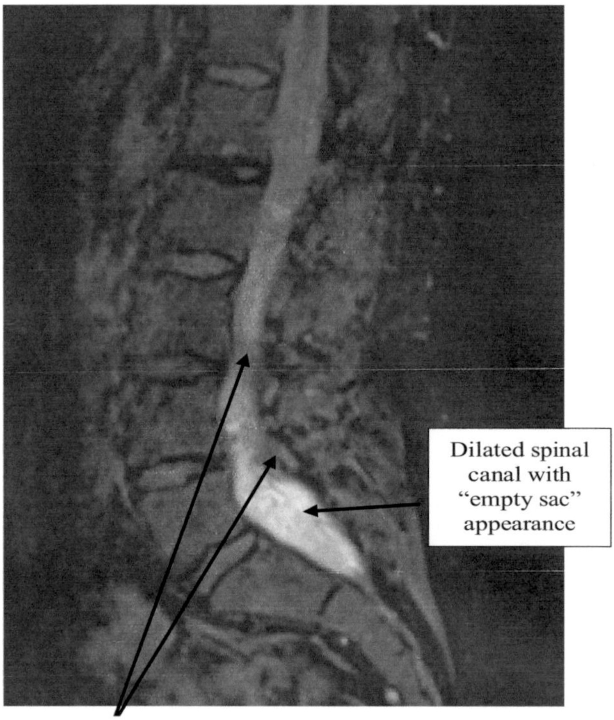

Multiple scarred AA masses are present. Dilation of the lower spinal canal is present due to a collagen deficient canal cover. Spinal fluid has collected in the lower canal. Patient is essentially bed bound, requires periodic catheterization to urinate, has lapses of memory, and has partial paralysis requiring a wheelchair to ambulate. Palliative, end-of-life care was required for relief and quality of life.

12. A STUDY OF THE EDS-AA CONNECTION

Once it was recognized that EDS is often connected to AA, an effort was made to gather some systematic data about these individuals. The purpose was to better recognize these individuals and develop a clinical profile of them. Within the Tennant Foundation a library of MRIs and clinical profiles of over 1000 persons with AA is maintained.

To obtain some systematic data on the EDS-AA connection, we put out a call by email in December of 2023 to our AA study group inviting persons with confirmed AA and EDS to voluntarily participate in a data collection study. Within less than two days we had 36 volunteer study participants. Dozens more individuals asked to be included, but this number (36) was convenient and could give us a base of information which is presented here. Each completed a lengthy questionnaire on their medical history, symptoms, and treatment. All provided us with whatever laboratory tests they had in their possession.

All study participants reported intractable (constant) pain and were in treatment with their local medical practitioners. Participants came from twenty different states, and three foreign countries. Several Tables are presented in this chapter to provide a medical profile and description of these individuals.

The findings are interesting in that the participants were almost all females. The high percentage of females versus males with EDS is well-documented in a number of reports. [8,9,72] A high percentage of study respondents were bed bound, due at least in part from difficulty with extremity function. These cases would be considered stage four or catastrophic AA cases.

All participants reported that their hypermobility began in childhood or teenage years. Almost all had their first episode of pain before age 20. Many made comments that their pain in childhood or as a teenager was simply thought to be "growing pains." A diagnosis of EDS wasn't given to most study participants until they were middle aged and had developed intractable pain.

The number of painful, pathologic conditions as well as the number of medical procedures that participants had undergone is striking. This group of 36 participants reported a total of 124 surgeries and 278 epidural injections. One can reasonably assume that the spine trauma of these interventions contributed to the development of AA.

The major pain relief medicinals were opioids and naltrexone. Ketorolac, methylprednisolone, and ketamine were the drugs most used for pain flares. The majority felt their treatment had either brought stability or slowed deterioration of their dual diseases. About a third felt their treatments were not working. Several mentioned they were undertreated.

Participants were asked to comment on any inappropriate or bizarre responses from physicians they had consulted for treatment. Several of the comments are presented in this chapter to make the point that there is still great ignorance about EDS. A goal of this handbook is to help erase this ignorance so persons with EDS can be identified and obtain the care they need.

A quick survey of the Tables emphasizes the extreme suffering and impairment of these participants. It is no wonder that suicide is common among persons with EDS and AA.

This is a small study from one source. Consequently, it cannot be assumed to necessarily represent all EDS and/or AA cases. The intent of the study was to obtain enough preliminary information to document the connection of EDS and AA and to signal the need to hopefully identify cases in their early stage.

Since, most participants in the study had hypermobility in childhood but weren't diagnosed with EDS until mid-life, an obvious conclusion is that a diagnosis of EDS in early life may have led to some preventive measures that would have prevented AA.

TABLE ONE SOME CHARACTERISTICS OF PERSONS WITH EDS AND AA N=36		
	No.	**%**
Females	34	94.4
Males	2	5.6
Bed bound most hours	13	36.1
Had infectious mononucleosis	9	20.0
Have autoimmune disease	10	27.8
Had complicated pregnancies	21	58.3
Symptoms worsened after a traumatic accident	8	22.2
Has intractable pain	36	100%

TABLE TWO KEY EVENTS BY AGE N = 36		
Age informed they were hypermobile	Range (yrs) Mean Age	3 to 56 18.6
Age diagnosed with hEDS	Range (yrs) Mean Age	28 to 84 48.7
Age of first pain episode	Range (yrs) Mean Age	3 to 52 12.9
Age of development of intractable pain	Range (yrs) Mean Age	10-79 42.6

All participants had constant, intractable pain at the time of study participation. They began intermittent or chronic pain in their teenage or young adult years and didn't develop intractable pain until much later.

TABLE THREE		
ANATOMIC PAIN SITES OF FIRST PAIN EPISODE N = 36		
FIRST PAIN EPISODE	**No.**	**%**
Headache	4	11.1
Shoulder/elbow	3	8.3
Hands/wrist	3	8.3
Foot/ankle	6	16.7
Back	6	16.7
Neck	5	13.9
Stomach	1	2.8
Hips	3	8.3
Knees	10	27.8
INTRACTABLE PAIN SITES		
Back/spine	28	77.8
Neck/spine	5	13.9
Non-spine site	3	8.3
Note: Some study participants reported that pain began in more than one anatomic site.		

TABLE FOUR PAINFUL CONDITIONS THAT PRECEDED OR ACCOMPANIED AA N = 36		
CONDITION	**No.**	**%**
Arthritis	36	100
Neuropathies	36	100
Migraine	27	75
Fibromyalgia	22	61.1
Irritable bowel	21	58.3
Temporal mandibular joint pain (TMJ)	20	55.6
Bursitis	18	50.0
Sciatica	17	47.2
Loss of teeth	17	47.2
Plantar fasciitis	15	41.7
Tendonitis	13	36.1
Chronic regional pain syndrome (CRPS)	9	25.0
Costochondritis	8	22.2
Pancreatitis	3	8.3
Every participant reported they had experienced multiple conditions.		

TABLE FIVE SPINAL CORD AND CANAL CONDITIONS REPORTED BY PARTICIPANTS WITH AA N = 36		
CONDITION	**No.**	**%**
Herniated discs	29	80.5
Tarlov cysts	18	50.0
Scoliosis	17	47.2
Spinal fluid leaks	15	41.7
Tethered cord	12	33.3
Cauda equina disorder	12	33.3
Chiari malformation	5	13.9
Persons in the study reported that these conditions occurred either before or simultaneously with AA. All participant reported more than a single condition.		

TABLE SIX PAIN TREATMENTS USED N = 36		
	No.	**%**
Opioids	26	72.2
Naltrexone alone	4	11.2
Naltrexone with an opioid	3	8.3
Used neither opioids nor naltrexone	3	8.3
Used ketorolac for pain flares	14	38.9
Used methylprednisolone or other corticosteroid for pain flares	9	25.0
Used ketamine for pain flares	5	13.9
Used anti-inflammatory medicinal	36	100.0
Perceived treatment to either stabilize or slow deterioration	23	63.9
Perceived treatment to be inadequate	13	36.1
Total No. of surgeries reported by all participants	124	
Total No. of epidural injections reported by all participants	278	

COMMENTS SAID TO STUDY PARTICIPANTS BY PHYSICIANS

- If you lose weight
- I'm crazy and anorexic
- Nothing is wrong with you
- Don't come back here
- You should go home and kill yourself because you'll be impossible to treat
- You just need to jog and eat more fruit
- You're born with it, so it doesn't cause any issues
- You just need to stress less
- There's nothing we can do for you
- You don't look like you're in that much pain
- A pain doctor gave me a signed contract that I needed to do her exercises and by 8 weeks, if I was compliant, I would not need opioids.
- All my pain is caused from my opioids (hyperalgesia)
- I need to exercise and eat better to feel better
- Cognitive behavior and physical therapy is all I need
- Just have to live with pain and accept it
- I don't have EDS and I shouldn't be taking so many opioids
- Well, you look great. You can't be in that much pain.
- You don't have autoimmunity.
- EDS doesn't cause pain.
- EDS is not disabling.
- You have hypermobility, not EDS.
- EDS cannot cause Tarlov Cysts or AA
- You don't probably have EDS. Even f you did, it wouldn't affect all this in your body
- If you will hang by your arms 1-2 times a day, your back pain will go away

- You don't have all these things wrong, you need anxiety medication
- Buck up, no one can have pain every moment of every day
- Have you tried removing gluten from your diet
- That EDS was useful and to my advantage because I wouldn't tighten up when I get older with arthritis and that I should work on stage fitting myself into a suitcase

13. THE CONNECTION BEGINS IN CHILDHOOD

EDS is an inherited disease of which the major pathologic impairment is a deficiency in either collagen production or metabolism. The result is that soft tissues such as muscle, nerves, tendons, fascia, and membranes are weakened. This condition is usually obvious in childhood. The first signs are "hypermobility," since the child can usually overextend some skin and joints.

Perhaps the best-known expression of gene-caused hypermobility is the lay term "double-joints." Another lay term is "flat feet." Children with EDS often find amusement with their body contortions and like to amuse their friends by showing off their ability to do such unusual anatomic positions as the "splits" or pull their leg or arm out of a socket.

Interestingly, the ability to overextend joints and do body contortions may make the child and teenager with EDS a great athlete, gymnast, or cheerleader as they can do body contortions and assume anatomic positions that other people can't do. Also, collagen deficiency in skin provides a smooth, most appealing look. Consequently, children and young adults with EDS may often be the good-looking, athletic persons we all admire. Unfortunately, the lack of collagen in tissue may lead one to believe the individual is "extra healthy" rather than have a body that is destined for disease, impairment, and premature death.

While some children and teenagers appear super healthy and athletic, some severe cases of EDS in childhood may suffer recurrent joint dislocations, bruising, falls, and fractures. Amazingly, some parents have been falsely accused of child abuse due to their children having EDS and showing the ravages of deficient collagen.

In the study described in the previous chapter plus other case reviews, we have learned that persons with the EDS-AA connection almost all had "growing pains" as a child or teenager. These symptoms were usually ignored and considered a normal variant. Some persons, however, had severe enough growing pains to require medication. Common painful symptoms in childhood include migraine and knee pain. In our arachnoiditis study project we have recently reviewed the cases of six children under the age of fourteen who have the EDS-AA connection. Undoubtedly, children in the past have developed the EDS-AA connection but were not recognized. Now that the connection is known, parents, physicians, and even teachers should know that the EDS-AA connection can start in childhood.

Children and teenagers with EDS are at risk of developing severe infections. Persons with EDS have a subnormal immune system. Consequently, the development of a severe infection such as infectious mononucleosis, meningitis, or pneumonia may often occur in children and teenagers with EDS. Severe infections in childhood and adolescence should be regarded as a risk factor for future autoimmunity and spine diseases.

A most pathetic and sad situation are the persons who reach middle age with EDS and have never been diagnosed. They may have developed AA before the diagnosis was even made. Without a current diagnosis these persons can become immobilized, bed-bound, and require catheters and diapers. They need assistance with eating and living. Some mentally adjust rather well to their plight and others long for the days of simple living and functioning. Loneliness is rampant as family and friends desert them. No wonder there is a high suicide rate among these individuals. The most potent palliative pain relief may be necessary.

Since children or teenagers with EDS are clearly at risk of developing severe medical complications including AA in adulthood, a preventive program should become part of their lives. They need a wholesome diet, exercises, and use of natural or herbal anti-inflammatories. Special stretching and muscle building exercises are well-described. [54] The Appendix lists the exercises we recommend for persons with AA and EDS. Aggressive medical treatment of any infection or trauma needs to be done. A key point to prevent AA is to recognize conditions that are known to be associated with active autoimmunity, and that autoimmunity can lead to AA. These diseases include fibromyalgia, constant migraines, neuropathy, thyroiditis, burning feet, mouth, or perineum, irritable bowel, and generalized pain. A particularly ominous sign is intervertebral disc degeneration and protrusion. Disc degeneration in a person with EDS represents active autoimmunity that needs to be suppressed in order to prevent AA.

TABLE

Some Possible Childhood/Teenage Risk Factors for the EDS-AA Connection

- ✓ Growing pains
- ✓ Headache
- ✓ Infectious mononucleosis
- ✓ Severe infection
- ✓ Joint dislocation
- ✓ Double-jointedness
- ✓ Can do body contortions such as the "splits"

End Stage EDS-AA Connection

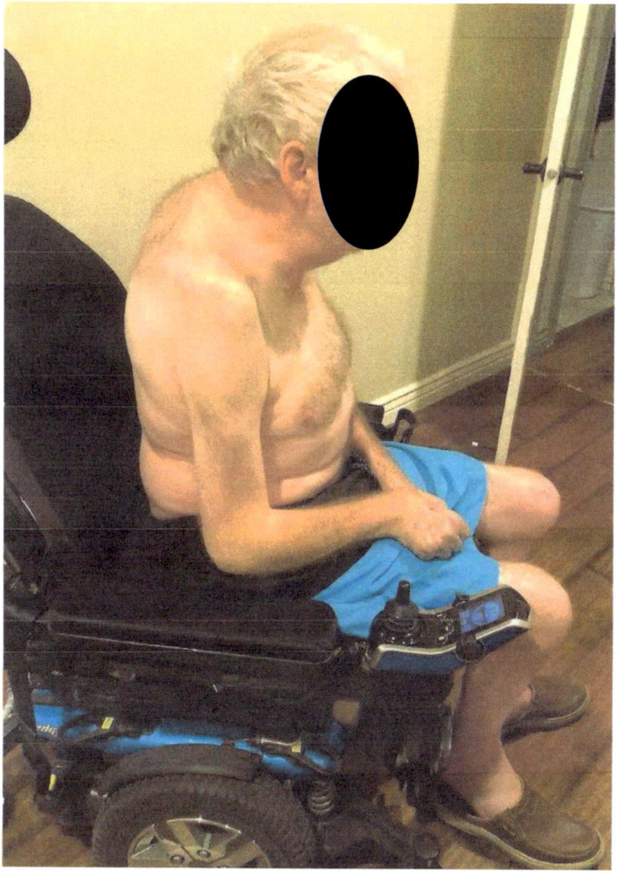

A disabled, bed-bound fifty-five-year-old man with EDS and AA. He was not diagnosed with either condition until he was in his early 50's. He gave no history of ongoing medical treatment with the exception of multiple spine surgeries.

14. EPSTEIN-BARR AUTOIMMUNITY-THE CONNECTION CATALYST?

Autoimmunity can be basically defined as a process or element inside the body that attacks and degenerates one's own tissues and causes disease and malfunctions. At the tissue or cellular site of an autoimmune attack or invasion, inflammation, tissue degeneration, and scarring will result when the tissue later attempts to heal. Pain and impairment of normal biologic functions at the tissue site will occur. This may involve the nerve and blood supply of the tissue-attack site. When scarring occurs, nerves may be either destroyed and/or entrapped. Permanent pain may result.

Parasitic reactivation and autoimmunity have been suspected to exist for at least three decades. Autoimmunity from active infections has been known since 1932 when Dr. Alvin Coburn determined that rheumatic heart disease and glomerulonephritis (kidney) may follow streptococcal throat infections. He was even the first to use the term "collagen disease" since he surmised that the streptococcal bacteria somehow damaged collagen in the heart. Autoimmunity following infectious mononucleosis has been known since the middle of the last century. In fact, this author reported a case of glomerulonephritis following infectious mononucleosis in 1968. EBV caught the world's attention in 1964 when Drs. Anthony Epstein and Yvonne Barr found the virus in a cancer known as Burkitt's lymphoma. Three years later the virus was determined to be the cause of infectious mononucleosis. The finding of the virus in a cancer clearly determined that EBV is more than an acute infection. It can enter the body, invade tissues, and cause cancer and other diseases.

In 2018, a seminal research study involving EBV changed the thinking about the virus and the care of intractable pain. [29,30] Dr. John Harley and his researchers at the VA Hospital and Children's Hospital in Cincinnati, Ohio unexpectedly announced a spectacular game-changing study on EBV. They found that an EBV protein (EBNA-2) interacted with genes that are associated with the development of multiple sclerosis, rheumatoid arthritis, inflammatory bowel disease, type 1 diabetes, juvenile arthritis, and celiac disease. All of these conditions are known to cause significant disability, impairments, and intractable pain. It also complimented some former blood studies which showed that patients with systemic lupus and rheumatoid arthritis demonstrated high levels of EBV IgG antibodies. Also, Dr. Harley's studies were funded by the US National Institute of Health, and his research paper had 14 co-authors. Simply put, this was a credible study involving many experts. Above all it forced all of us to take notice, change direction, and take EBV autoimmunity and tissue invasion very seriously.

To add to Dr. Harley's motivating work, Dr. Kjetil Bjornevik and ten colleagues later published in 2022 a highly complementary report in Science. It showed that 955 active-duty military young adults with multiple sclerosis had high levels of EBV IgG antibodies. [6] Other reports and papers since the Harley and Bjornevik studies support the notion that EBV may produce an autoimmune disease and/or invade tissues and cause some cancers and neurologic diseases. [33,74]

Given Dr. Harley's studies, it was clearly apparent that AA needs to be researched for EBV autoimmunity. Multiple sclerosis is a spinal cord inflammatory disease and so is AA. Some persons with AA have multiple sclerosis, consequently, we set out to immediately start collecting antibody tests from persons with AA. At the time this book is being written, we have now reviewed EBV-IgG antibody tests in over 150 persons with MRI-documented AA. Every case, including those who have EDS, has shown high (above laboratory normal range) of IgG antibodies which are now regarded as markers for EBV autoimmunity. This seeming universal finding in confirmed AA cases has compelled us to believe that EBV autoimmunity either causes or accelerates the development of AA. Since EBV may be a cause or catalyst for the EDS-AA connection, a summary of EBV and its pathologic machinations are summarized here.

EBV is a natural, lifelong parasite in the human body. It usually enters the body before one is two years old. When it enters the body it may cause a cold, sinusitis, or bronchitis, and likely go unnoticed. After the initial infection, EBV settles into one's lymphocytes (beta class) to remain for life. Under normal physiologic circumstances it is "latent" or "dormant" and does no harm. Over 95% of adults will test negative for IgM antibodies and show low levels of IgG antibodies indicating they have previously, not currently, had an active infection. Laboratories now realize the importance of EBV and have developed normal ranges for IgM and IgG antibodies. These tests now give the medical practitioner the ability to help determine if their patients have EBV reactivation, autoimmunity, and possibly tissue invasion.

EBV is a member of the herpes virus (#4) family which includes the other herpes viruses and cytomegalovirus. Even though the herpes viruses are natural parasites that live dormant in our lymphocytes, they are known as "opportunistic." This means that during times of stress the virus may reactivate and produce an autoimmune disorder or replicate and invade tissues outside lymphocytes. To illustrate, some other strains (labialis zoster, simplex) of the herpes virus family may reactivate during times of stress and produce a small ulcer (canker sore) on the lip, or blister-type lesions on the genitalia. Herpes zoster causes a skin eruption (shingles) along nerve routes most commonly on the chest, back, or legs.

EBV remains harmless in our lymphocytes unless there is excess stress on the body that renders the lymphocyte's normal immune protection system unable to suppress the virus. [43] Stress can be trauma, infection, malnutrition, or even psychological. For example, many persons with the EDS-AA connection report disease deterioration following an auto accident or other trauma including medical procedures. When this occurs, the latent virus takes this opportunity to reactivate and begin to replicate itself. Lymphocytes chronically infected with activated EBV may enter any number of tissues and even cross the blood brain barrier to enter the spinal cord and brain tissues. The virus may undergo a lytic or replication phase to permanently infect tissues outside the lymphocyte. This includes glial cells in the brain and spinal cord.[37,38,40,74] Inflammation, adhesions, and tissue damage in the brain may be the result. EBV autoimmunity and/or tissue invasion of the central nervous system has to now be a strong consideration as a cause of intractable pain. EBV autoimmunity or invasion of tissues may cause inflammation which may lead to the destruction of neurotransmitter-receptor systems that normally control or shut down pain so that it doesn't become constant and intractable.

During reactivation EBV may produce a toxic substance, autoantibody, or other autoimmune mechanism that can attack and injure tissues throughout the body. [33,37,38,71] Although the precise mechanism is unclear, this process or disease is now called "EBV Autoimmunity." Until now EBV autoimmunity has not been taken seriously. Given EBV's ability to produce cancer, some autoimmune diseases, and multiple sclerosis, it is not unreasonable to believe it is a causative catalyst of the EDS-AA connection. Our studies which show elevated IgG antibodies in confirmed AA cases, support this view.

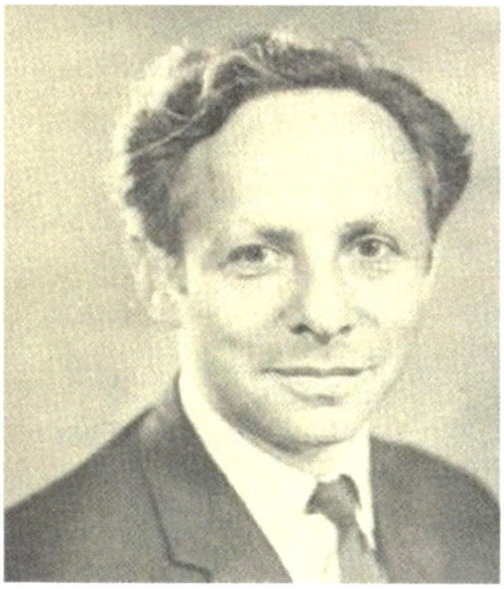

Dr. Anthony Epstein

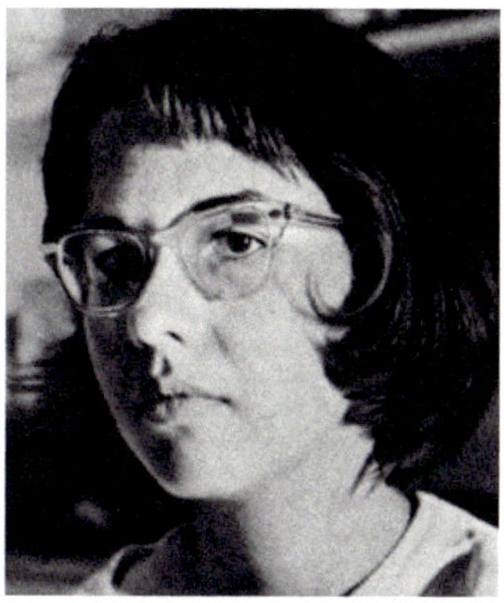

Dr. Yvonne Barr

In 1964 Drs. Epstein and Barr discovered the virus in a cancer called Burkitt's lymphoma. The virus is of the herpes class and now bears their names (Epstein-Barr). About three years after their discovery the virus was found to be the cause of infectious mononucleosis. Their discovery of the virus in a cancer proved that the virus under some circumstances can invade tissues, and cause disease.

15. TREATMENT OF THE CONNECTION

Once EDS and AA are clinically present treatment is primarily directed at AA. EDS is a genetic disease, so it does not have a specific treatment. Therapeutic measures are directed at the many symptoms and complications caused by EDS. Recently a superb book entitled "Symptomatic: The Symptom-Based Handbook for Ehlers-Danlos Syndromes and Hypermobility Spectrum Disorders" was published to assist medical practitioners who treat patients with EDS. It is edited by Drs. Claire Francomano, Alan Hakim, Lansdale Henderson, and Fraser Henderson, all internationally known EDS experts, along with over five dozen specialists who are authorities in specialized clinical complications of EDS. This book describes symptoms and treatments for every aspect of EDS, and it is highly recommended as a desk-top, quick reference to any medical practitioner who treats EDS patients. I wish to add here that the pain of EDS patients may be intractable, severe, and disabling due to small fiber neuropathy and spinal inflammatory conditions. The drugs needed to adequately treat the intractable pain of EDS patients may often require potent drugs that carry an overdose and abuse risk and may carry a labeled warning and/or be subject to various restrictions and guidelines. The severity of pain in EDS almost always justifies use of such drugs including opioids, benzodiazepines, and amphetamine derivatives. There is a concept in intractable and palliative pain care known as "Maximal Medical Pain Relief." It is patterned after the Brompton Cocktail made famous in the last century as the pain treatment necessary for the severest of pain. A detailed description of the Brompton Cocktail and its modern version is in the Appendix.

At this time, the author is reviewing the use of some specific hormones and peptides in EDS. Although their use appears promising, it is too early to recommend their general use.

A three-component medical protocol is recommended for treatment of AA. The first component is suppression of autoimmunity and inflammation. The second component is to rebuild and regenerate damaged cauda equina nerves and the arachnoid membrane. Pain relief is the third component. Relief is necessary so the person with AA can physically and mentally function not just to carry out activities of daily living but to participate in the dietary and physical measures necessary to control AA. Below is a brief description of each component. A three-component starting protocol (Day One) is in the Appendix.

Some popular medicinals are listed in each component to assist patients, families, and medical practitioners in building an effective program to control AA. It is emphasized that the medicinals suggested here have not been verified or substantiated by controlled studies but have emerged as "popular" agents. No assurance or probabilities of effectiveness can, therefore, be given. It is to be emphasized that in our clinical reviews and studies the three component treatment is much more effective in mild or moderate rather than in severe and catastrophic cases.

1. Component One – Suppression of Inflammation and Autoimmunity

   Some popular medicinals include ketorolac, methylprednisolone, diclofenac, dexamethasone, luteolin, quercetin, and curcumin.

2. Component Two - Rebuild and Regenerate Damaged Tissues

   Cauda equina nerves and arachnoid membrane which have been injured by inflammation and/or autoimmunity must be regenerated and healed to reduce pain and neurologic impairments. Popular medicinals include colostrum, dehydroepiandrosterone (DHEA), human chorionic gonadotropin (HCG), polypeptides, and nandrolone. Trials of electro microcurrents and/or electromagnetic energy therapy, protein-anti-inflammatory diet, and select physical measures are highly recommended (See Appendix).

3. Component Three – Pain Control

   Medicinals to relieve pain are necessary for both physical and mental functioning. AA is such a devastating and life-shortening disease that high dosages of pain relievers are justified in severe and catastrophic cases. Popular medicinals include low dose naltrexone, opioids, palmitoylethanolamide (PEA), ketamine, medical marijuana, kratom, and oxytocin. A neuropathic agent such as gabapentin, pregabalin, clonazepam and an amphetamine derivative such as dextroamphetamine or methylphenidate may also be required for effective pain relief.

Intractable pain occurs in almost all persons with AA. It is defined as constant pain that produces cardiovascular, endocrine, immunologic, and metabolic complications. The basic cause is believed to be destruction and dysfunction of receptor-neurotransmitter systems in the central nervous system.

These become too impaired and damaged to shut down pain, so it becomes constant. The mechanism whereby neurotransmitters and receptor systems become damaged begins with inflammation in glial cells .[50,51] Just as inflammation in the skin (cellulitis) may spread, glial cells may spread inflammation to surrounding tissue causing destruction and scarring. Brain scans of persons with intractable pain may show small, scarred areas. Effective anti-inflammatory treatment in AA is directed not just at inflammation in the lower spinal canal but at inflammation in the brain.[22,35,44,45] Pain relief may require "maximal medical treatment" which is a regimen patterned after the famous Brompton Cocktail. It is in the Appendix. An implanted electrical spinal stimulator or opioid infusion device may be justified and effective in severe and catastrophic cases of AA.

The three-component medical protocol listed here should be supported by some specific dietary and physical measures. A daily protein, anti-inflammatory diet is recommended along with certain dietary supplements such as vitamins C, D, B-12 with the minerals magnesium, zinc, or selenium. These supplements have been shown to help suppress Epstein-Barr reactivation as well as help rebuild tissue.[43] A trial with a collagen supplement is recommended. Although defective metabolism and production of collagen is present in persons with EDS, many persons with EDS and AA feel that collagen supplements are helpful.

Three basic types of physical measures are highly recommended for persons with AA and EDS. One is spinal fluid flow exercises. [71] AA is a mass or masses in the lower spinal canal which blocks and interrupts the flow of spinal fluid. Rocking in a chair, gently bouncing on a trampoline, walking with arm swings, and deep breathing, are all positive measures that may enhance spinal fluid flow. Persons with AA who have blurred vision, vertigo, headache, and mental aberrations may benefit from acetazolamide. The second group of physical measures is done primarily to maintain physical functioning of the feet, legs, arms which may weaken and even become partially or totally paralyzed to the point that one needs a cane, walker, or wheelchair. Basic extremity protection and maintenance measures include walking, stretching, and light weightlifting. Thirdly, daily water soaking is recommended. Some specific dietary and physical measures are in the Appendix.

It is to be emphasized that neither EDS nor AA are curable diseases. Long-term treatment protocols and regimens need to be developed individually for each person with assistance and input from family members. Patients are constantly bombarded with offers of a one-time, short-term "fix" or "magic bullet." This author considers these to be measures that may be tried after a patient is stabilized on a 3-component medical protocol with supportive dietary and physical measures.

16. OPPORTUNITIES FOR PREVENTION

The disease combination of EDS and AA is tragic. Persons with both diseases suffer medically, mentally, and socially. Families must struggle financially and emotionally to deal with the connection. Pain, suffering, and a premature death are common. No data exists on suicide among connection cases, but it is clearly significant. Prevention of the connection is an obvious necessity. But is prevention possible? Yes, the prevention of the connection is clearly doable. EDS is an inherited or genetic condition that can't be prevented. The key is to prevent the development of AA. There are several ways to do this, and all families of a child with EDS must know the risk as well as adults with EDS regardless of their age.

First, EDS needs to be recognized in childhood or teenage years. The child with double joints who can contort their bodies must be viewed with the serious realization of what may happen in adulthood. No longer can these children be viewed with either amazement or aggrandizement if they have good looks and athleticism. Children who demonstrate or complain of headaches, joint pain, growing pains, or have a severe infection need to be evaluated for the possibility of EDS.

Children with EDS who can voluntarily extend or dislocate an arm or leg or twist their body into a contortion, should be educated and reprimanded to never do these movements. It is possible that every over-extension or contortion adds "insult to injury." Since the person with EDS already has deficient collagen strands in their tissues, every over-extension and contortion simply puts more strain and damage to the deficient collagen. The risk for infections, neuropathies, and pain just went up!!

Healthy exercises such as walking and swimming are essential. A balanced diet of protein, fat, and carbohydrates should be standard. Vitamin and mineral supplements are advised. The old "one a day" vitamin-mineral tab or cap is a good place to start. Diet doesn't have to be terribly restrictive. It needs to have three main components. First, an adequate daily intake of protein is essential. Protein foods are mainly seafood, beef, pork, poultry, and eggs. Second, a daily intake of some anti-inflammatory vegetables and fruits is essential. Lastly, sugars (carbohydrates) have to be restricted. Parasitic viruses such as Epstein-Barr thrive on high blood sugars. As described in the chapter on EBV, new research indicates that parasitic viruses may reactivate and create autoimmunity. All persons with EDS have to take heed of this new information. Although many authorities believe that collagen supplements are ineffective due to defective genetic collagen production in EDS, many persons with EDS and their medical practitioners, however, recommend them. To date, I know of no harm that has been done to persons with EDS who take collagen supplements, and a trial of four to six weeks to see some physiologic improvement is worth the attempt.

A popular and growing trend is to provide herbal or natural anti-inflammatory agents and low doses of anabolic (growth) hormones to teenagers and young adults with EDS. Popular herbal agents include turmeric, luteolin, quercetin, and astragalus. Popular hormones are colostrum, deer antler velvet, and dehydroepiandrosterone (DHEA). Colostrum and deer antler velvet contain low dosages of a number of natural growth hormones. None of these have scientific studies to recommend them. Their use is strictly a hope to prevent tissue degeneration and future tragedy. The author knows some persons with EDS who have taken colostrum and/or natural or herbal agents for several years and have remained quite well and functional now that they are seventy plus years of age.

Perhaps the best opportunity to prevent AA is to be aware that any person with EDS who has herniated discs, spinal fluid leaks, or Tarlov cysts are at very high risk of developing AA. These conditions, particularly if there is no history of trauma, should arise suspicion that an autoimmune-inflammatory disorder may be present. As described in chapter 14, Epstein-Barr autoimmunity should be a serious consideration.

Based on the author's experience and study, persons with EDS should avoid spinal surgery, injections, and spinal taps unless a medical urgency calls for them. Unfortunately, persons with EDS have a collagen deficiency, so any invasive spinal intervention may foster the development of destructive inflammation and adhesion formation within the spinal canal.

Today, all persons with EDS need to know as early as possible if they are developing a rheumatic disease or autoimmunity. This requires periodic (e.g., yearly) blood tests for inflammatory and autoimmune markers. A new set of inflammatory markers are called cytokines and interleukins.

All major laboratories offer interleukin panels, and persons with EDS need one at least yearly. Any elevation calls for anti-inflammatory measures. A number (and growing) of autoimmune markers are now available. These include the old standards such as the antinuclear autoantibody (ANA), and tests for rheumatoid arthritis and systemic lupus markers. Today, EBV antibodies are recommended as early research is progressively suggesting that EBV reactivation and autoimmunity puts one at elevated risk of AA. If a person with EDS has blood indicators of inflammation and/or autoimmunity, they need to immediately start building a therapeutic program to suppress inflammation and autoimmunity to prevent AA.

SUMMARY

AA has long been known to be a disease of great misery, incapacitation, and early death. It was known as a "devil's disease" in the 1800's. Thanks to antibiotic therapy for syphilis and tuberculosis and the MRI which eliminated the use of toxic myelogram dyes, AA essentially disappeared and was classified as a rare disease in the last half of the past century. For reasons that are not fully understood, AA, however, began to clinically reappear in the early years of this century.

Surprisingly, at least 30 to 50 % of confirmed AA cases have EDS. EDS is an inherited disease that has two characteristics which make the individual prone to develop AA: (1) collagen deficiency and (2) immune deficiency. Persons with both EDS and AA may be extremely ill with intractable pain and multiple neurologic impairments. Although no specific treatment is available for either disease, a three-component medical protocol is recommended for AA that (1) suppresses inflammation and autoimmunity, (2) regenerates or rebuilds the cauda equina and arachnoid membrane, and (3) relieves pain.

There are opportunities to prevent the development of the EDS-AA connection. The first is to recognize the child or teenager who has EDS. This young individual may benefit from a healthy diet, maintenance of muscular and neurologic strength and function, and suppression of inflammation. AA is always preceded by an inflammatory condition of the spine, especially herniated discs. Aggressive control of spinal inflammation may prevent the development of AA.

At this time, there is growing evidence that EBV autoimmunity is a causative or catalytic factor in the development of AA. It is possible that AA can be prevented or ameliorated if EBV reactivation and autoimmunity is suppressed.

The EDS-AA connection is a tragic occurrence. It can easily be recognized by all concerned parties. In most cases AA can be prevented, but if the connection does develop, humanitarian treatment can at least ameliorate the connection's multiple pathologic complications, and give the person some quality of life.

APPENDIX

a. Diagnostic Screen for Hypermobile Spectrum Disorder and Collagen Deficiency Diseases

	Questions for Collagen Deficiency Determination	Y	N
1	Do you bruise easily?		
2	Do your legs, knees, or ankles feel weak at times?		
3	Do you lose your balance or fall frequently?		
4	Are your wounds slow to heal?		
5	Have you lost teeth or had a lot of dental work?		
6	Have you developed herniated or slipped discs without heavy lifting or trauma?		
7	Do you have flat feet or fallen arches?		
8	Do you have burning sensations of feet, mouth, or groin area?		
9	Do you easily sprain your back, arms, or legs with overexertion?		
10	Do you have stomach or bowel problems that require regular antacids, probiotics, or laxatives?		
11	Do you have any genetic deformities of feet, toes, mouth, or hands?		
12	As a child or teenager did you get injured too easily to play sports or do other physical activities?		
13	As a child or teenager did you have growing pains or knee pains?		
14	Have you ever dislocated a joint such as your elbow, shoulder, knee, or hip?		
15	Females: Did you have complications with pregnancy or delivery?		
16	Do you have relatives with life-long skeletal deformities or severe pain?		
This questionnaire has been developed by the author to help determine if a patient has a hypermobile spectrum disorder, Marfan Syndrome, or other collagen deficiency disease.			

Special Note: If half the questions are answered yes, further evaluation including tests for autoimmunity and inflammation are warranted.

b. Stages and Categorization of Adhesive Arachnoiditis Severity

Adhesive arachnoiditis (AA) is a progressive, inflammatory disease that may pass through stages. The category and stages are mainly determined by the number of cauda equina nerves that are inflamed, entrapped, and scarred inside the lumbar-sacral spinal canal. Below are the four stages and categories of AA.

□ Mild - Stage One

	A	Extremities: full range of motion, strength, extension
	B	No urinary or central* symptoms
	C	Normal ambulation
	D	Intermittent pain. Non-opioid management is sufficient.

□ Moderate - Stage Two

	A	Extremities: full range of motion, strength, extension
	B	Some urinary, gastrointestinal tract, and/or central symptoms
	C	Normal ambulation
	D	Constant pain, but manageable with low dose or intermittent opioids

□ Severe - Stage Three

	A	Extremities: some deficiency in range of motion, strength, or extension
	B	Has significant urinary, gastrointestinal tract, and/or central symptoms
	C	Ambulates with assistance (cane, walker, wheelchair)
	D	Severe constant pain that requires daily opioids

□ Catastrophic - Stage Four

	A	Extremities: significant deficiencies in range of motion, strength, or extension
	B	Significant urinary, gastrointestinal tract, or central symptoms
	C	Bed bound some of each day
	D	Ambulation requires assistance
	E	Severe intractable pain that requires palliative care and daily potent opioids

Notes on Interpretation: *Central refers to headaches, eye/ear/nasal symptoms such as blurred vision, tinnitus, vertigo, or nasal dripping. MRI findings do not necessarily correlate with staging although the severe and catastrophic categories usually show one or more of these findings: dense scarring of cauda equina nerve clumps, multiple clumps, lower spinal canal distension (empty sac), peripheralization, and/or calcification.

Categories can overlap. Mild and moderate categories have the best potential for amelioration. A three-component medical protocol (1. Suppression of inflammation; 2. Tissue rebuilding and regeneration; 3. Pain relief) with supporting diet and exercises is recommended for stages one, two, and three. Stage four/catastrophic requires palliative care for intractable pain.

An implanted electrical stimulator or opioid infusion device may be necessary for palliative care.

c. *Dietary Measures for Adhesive Arachnoiditis*

AA is a progressive inflammatory disease. The diet is intended to help reduce pain by the intake of anti-inflammatory food and regeneration of inflamed tissue. It is also intended to help prevent Epstein Barr Virus (EBV) reactivation.

A. Daily Multivitamin-Mineral Tab/Cap

B. Daily Vitamin: C (2000 to 4000 mg a day)

C. Daily Selenium, Magnesium, or Zinc

D. Collagen Supplement

E. Options : Vitamins B-12, D-3, K-2, E

F. Foods and Drinks

1. Each day: eat one or more of these protein foods: beef, lamb, pork, poultry (chicken, turkey), seafood (fish, shrimp, crab), cottage cheese, eggs

2. Each day: eat some vegetables and/or fruits

3. Stop drinks that contain regular sugar (carbohydrates) including fruit juices and soft drinks

4. Restrict sugars and starches known as carbohydrates (e.g., breads, candy, pastries, pasta)

d. Physical Exercises for Adhesive Arachnoiditis (AA)

Essential Physical Exercises: Certain, specific exercises are recommended to help free cauda equina nerves from entrapment, maintain neurologic functions, and enhance spinal fluid flow. Daily walks are considered essential to maintain function and prevent paralysis.

Exercises for Spinal Fluid Flow Enhancement

1. Rocking chair – 5 to 10 minutes
2. Walking or gentle bouncing on a trampoline – 3 to 5 minutes
3. Deep breathing – hold each breath for 5-10 seconds
4. Arm swings while walking

Free Nerves and Maintain Functions

1. Stretch arms straight up and hold for 5-10 seconds
2. While standing, raise one knee and leg at a time and hold for 5-10 seconds
3. Flex your ankle and foot 5-10 times. Can repeat several times a day.
4. Walk with arms swings only as far as energy will allow. Don't overdue.
5. Lift three-to-four-pound weights. Do no more than 5 lifts at a time.
6. Flex and hold neck in both forward and backward positions. Hold for 5 to 10 seconds.
7. Stand straight up with legs together. Look slightly upward for 10 seconds ("military attention").

Major Message

1. One doesn't have to do every exercise. Select one or two that you will do every day. You can do some of the stretching exercises several times a day.
2. Essential: Persons with AA should take at least two short walks a day (at least 100 feet) to maintain leg and foot function.

e. Starting Three-Component Medical Protocol for Mri-Documented Cases Of AA

This protocol is suggested as starting medical treatment for ambulatory, neurologically intact persons who have a typical history, symptoms, and MRI-documentation of AA.

COMPONENT ONE: Suppression of Inflammation and Autoimmunity

1. Ketorolac (Toradol®) 20-30 mg (oral or injection) in home or practitioner's office every 1 to 2 weeks
2. Methylprednisolone 4 mg or dexamethasone 0.5 mg oral, 1 to 2 days a week

   Options or add-ons:
   a. Quercetin, luteolin, curcumin, andrographis
   b. Suppression of viral reactivation (Epstein-Barr or other): vitamin C, lysine, zinc, or selenium

COMPONENT TWO: Regeneration of Cauda Equina Nerves and Arachnoid Membrane

1. Pentoxifylline (Trental®), 400 mg, 2 to 3 times a day with vitamin E, 800 to 1000 mg a day
2. Add a regeneration hormone and/or peptide within one to ten days. Use 3 to 4 days a week.
   a. Regeneration hormones (HCG, colostrum, DHEA, nandrolone)
   b. *Regeneration peptides (BPC-157, KPV, thymosin beta)

COMPONENT THREE: Relief of Pain

1. Start low dose naltrexone (LDN) 0.5 to 1.0 mg twice a day or (a) a low dose opioid (buprenorphine, codeine, tramadol) or (b) remain on opioid or other pain reliever used prior to this protocol.

2. Neuropathic agent: Choice of gabapentin, pregabalin, clonazepam, carisoprodol. Leave on any effective agent used prior to this protocol.

   Options or Add-ons for Flare Pain: palmitoylethanolamide (PEA), marijuana, kratom, ketamine, oxytocin

Notes on Protocol Usage:

1. The patient should remain on any medication for pain, sleep, and other symptoms that were effectively being treated prior to starting this protocol.

2. This protocol can possibly be enhanced by a daily protein, anti-inflammatory diet. Physical measures such walking, stretching, and deep breathing should be done daily. Microcurrent administration is highly recommended.

3. This protocol is not applicable to persons with AA who are non-ambulatory, bed-bound, suffer intractable pain, and have neurologic impairment of bladder or bowel. Palliative care is recommended in this situation.

4. *Ketorolac and methylprednisolone are deemed essential in the treatment of AA. They are used intermittently at low doses to prevent side effects.

Other corticosteroids (e.g. prednisone, hydrocortisone) are not usually effective due to their inability to cross the blood brain barrier, enter spinal fluid, and attach to specific receptors in the central nervous system.

5. Abbreviations
    a. HCG is human chorionic gonadotropin
    b. DHEA is dehydroepiandrosterone
    c. BPC is Body Protection Compound
    d. KPV is lysine, proline, valine

f. Maximal Medical Treatment for Palliative Pain Care

There is a maximal medical treatment for palliative pain care that dates to the Brompton Hospital in London, England in 1895. The "Brompton Cocktail" was a multi-drug liquid formulation. This formulation was used extensively for palliative pain care in the last century when pharmaceutical companies designed and marketed oral agents to conveniently substitute for a liquid formation.

Major Message: Science in recent years has shown why the Brompton cocktail "worked" so well. It simultaneously activates the three major neurotransmitter-receptor systems in the brain and spinal cord that relieve severe pain. These are the endocrine, dopamine, and gamma amino butyric acid (GABA) neurotransmitter-receptor systems.

Table Showing Brompton Cocktail Ingredients and Today's Medicinals Substitutes

Target Neurotransmitter-receptor System	Brompton Cocktail	Contemporary Agents
Endorphin	Morphine	Methadone, morphine, fentanyl, oxycodone, hydromorphone
Dopamine/norepinephrine	Cocaine	Methylphenidate, dextroamphetamine, amphetamine salts (Adderall®), phentermine
Gamma amino butyric acid (GABA)	Alcohol, chloroform	Diazepam, clonazepam, gabapentin, pregabalin, carisoprodol
Anti-inflammatory*	Aspirin	Ketorolac, methylprednisolone, dexamethasone, diclofenac

Clinical Need: Maximal medical treatment may be required for the severity of intractable pain produced by such clinical entities as the dual combination of EDS-AA.

*Aspirin was given but not usually in the cocktail.

g. *Blood Tests for Epstein-Barr Virus Reactivation and Autoimmunity*

The purpose of Epstein-Barr-Virus (EBV IgG antibody) tests is to determine if viral reactivation and autoimmunity is present in persons with an intractable pain condition such as AA or EDS. IgM antibody, polymerase chain reaction (PCR), and DNA analysis are for acute infection and not for reactivation or autoimmunity. IgG tests must be quantitative not simply positive or negative.

<u>The EBV IgG Antibody Tests to Help Determine Autoimmunity are:</u>

1. EBV nuclear antigen IgG antibody (abbreviated EBNA)
2. EBV viral capsid IgG antibody (abbreviated VCA)

These two tests, when above normal laboratory levels, suggest that past EBV reactivation has occurred, and that autoimmunity is present.

<u>The EBV IgG Antibody Test for Reactivation</u>

Early Epstein-Barr nuclear antigen IgG antibody (abbreviated EA-EBNA)

<u>SUMMARY:</u> VCA and EBNA IgG antibodies are markers of probable autoimmunity. If elevated and there is the clinical presence of disorders known to be associated with autoimmunity such as fibromyalgia, neuropathies, thyroiditis, burning mouth, rheumatic diseases, and irritable bowel, a clinical diagnosis of EBV autoimmunity is justified. A high IgG early EBNA indicates current reactivation.

GLOSSARY OF TERMS

Adhesive Arachnoiditis: An intraspinal canal inflammatory disorder in which a clump or mass of cauda equina nerves are glued by adhesions to the arachnoid-dural covering of the spinal canal.

Adhesive arachnoiditis ossification: This term has been applied to cases that show calcification in the clump or mass of AA.

Arachnoiditis-non-adhesive: Inflammation of the arachnoid layer of the spinal canal covering (meninges) without any nerves adhered to it. This condition cannot specifically be identified by MRI. It is a clinical diagnosis based on signs, symptoms, and laboratory tests.

Axial view: "Toe-to-Head" view or images of the cauda equina and spinal canal. It is a cross section or pictorial "slice" of the spinal canal.

Autoimmunity: A disease process or element in the body that attacks and destroys tissue.

Bioelectricity: The electricity formed in tissue that fosters metabolism, muscular movement, and neurologic functions.

Canal distortion: The normal circular contour of the spinal canal has lost its normal shape due to some pathologic process such as fibrosis, scarring, or loss of tensile strength.

Cauda equina: About two dozen nerves that emanate from the spinal cord at the level of thoracic 12(T-12) or lumbar 1 (L-1) vertebrae and are suspended in spinal fluid. The term nerve roots is often applied rather than nerves.

Chronic Pain: A pain that persists longer than the usual healing time of about ninety days.

Circular contour: Cauda equina nerves normally appear circular on the axial view of an MRI. Loss of circular contour represents edema, inflammation, or degeneration.

Clumping or coalescence: Multiple cauda equina nerves have joined together due to inflammation and adhesion formation.

Collagen: A strong fibrous insoluble protein found in the dermis, tendons, ligaments, deep fascia, bone, cartilage, nerves, and membranes.

Connective Tissue Disorder: A genetic disease in which collagen in tissues is deficient and weakens the tissues which may result in inflammation, adhesions, scarring, and pain.

Contrast: The ability to distinguish spinal fluid by white coloring from solid tissue which shows as varying shades of gray. This may be accomplished with intravenous dye or with high resolution imaging.

Corticoid or Corticosteroid: A pharmaceutical that is chemically related to cortisone.

Disorganization: Severe displacement with gross distortion of the normal cauda equina nerve pattern.

Displacement: One or more cauda equina nerves are moved or located in an abnormal position on axial (toe-to-head) MRI images.

Dormant: State in which a parasitic virus is in tissues but inactive and not causing any pathologic complications.

Ehlers-Danlos Syndrome (EDS): A genetic collagen deficient, connective tissue disorder named after two physicians who first described the condition. The most common form is hypermobile.

Empty sac: The lower lumbar and/or sacral spinal canal is dilated with no sign of nerve roots passing through the interior of the canal. The cause is nerve roots being completely adhered and attached to the inside of the spinal canal covering rather than be free floating in the spinal fluid.

Epidural Injection: An injection given in the space just above the spinal canal.

Epstein Barr Virus: A virus of the herpes class that is normally an innocuous human parasite but may activate and produce an autoimmune disorder and a number of pathologic conditions including some cancers and neurologic diseases. Named after the scientists who discovered the virus in a cancer known as Burkitt's lymphoma.

Failed Back Surgery Syndrome: Condition assigned to persons who had spine surgery that failed to relieve the pain for which surgery was done.

Herb: A medicinal that comes from a plant or botanical.

Hypermobile: The ability to extend or over-extend skin and joints beyond normal range.

Hypermobile Spectrum Disorder: A group of about a dozen, rare genetic collagen deficient, connective tissue conditions that are related to hypermobile EDS.

Inflammation: Tissue that is red, hot, degenerating, and causes pain and neurologic impairments.

Intractable Pain: Constant, incurable pain that may produce cardiovascular, respiratory, endocrine, and metabolic complications.

Latent Phase: A state after initial infection when a virus is quiet, silent, and harmless. Same meaning as dormant.

Lumbar levels: There are five lumbar vertebrae levels being designated L1 through L5 with L1 being the topmost vertebrae.

Lumbar Spine: A lower back section of the spine consisting of five lumbar vertebrae levels being designated L1 through L5 with L1 being the topmost vertebrae.

Lytic Phase: Period in which a virus is multiplying or replicating by dividing itself.

Marfan Syndrome: A hereditary disorder of connective tissue, bones, muscles, ligaments, and skeletal structures. It is characterized by a tall lean body with long fingers, toes, joint flexibility, and flat feet.

Meninges: This is the covering of the brain and upper spinal canal consisting of three layers: dura, arachnoid, and pia mater. In the lumbar-sacral region of the spine, the covering primarily consists of an inside layer, the arachnoid, and an outer layer, dura. The word “covering” is preferentially used in this book rather than meninges or theca to simplify understanding.

Natural: A medicinal that is made in the human body.

Peripheralization: Cauda equina nerves have moved to the periphery of the spinal canal and are adhered by adhesions to the inside of the spinal canal cover. This finding is often called "empty sac" as the canal may look empty on both axial and lateral MRI views.

Precursor: An antecedent medical condition that leads to another or a chemical substance that makes another by metabolism.

Reactivation: Refers to a virus that is usually dormant or latent and starts to divide and propagate producing active infection and/or an autoimmune state.

Receptor: A molecular tissue site composed of protein which receives a neurotransmitter or biochemical and then creates some function.

Sagittal View: This is the side or lateral MRI view of the spine.

Seepage: Spinal fluid that has leaked or seeped into tissues outside the spinal canal. Contrast MRI imaging shows spinal fluid as white.

Skin channels: Spinal fluid has seeped through the arachnoid-dural cover of the spinal canal and worked its way to the skin surface. In this process tracks or channels between the spine and skin surface are formed.

Spacing: This refers to the normal space between cauda equina nerves as seen on axial MRI images. The space appears as white between gray or black nerve roots. Spacing disappears with nerve enlargement or coalescence.

Spinal canal: Also known as the thecal sac. The spinal canal is a structure like a closed pipe that carries the spinal fluid. The fluid is primarily produced in the brain and flows down the canal on one side and flows back up to the brain to be diverted into lymph nodes and the general blood and lymphatic systems. The word canal is preferentially used here to simplify understanding.

Spinal Tap: A puncture of the spinal canal to either place a substance inside the canal or withdraw fluid.

Spine: Refers to the entire spine including vertebrae, intervertebral discs, spinal canal, cord inside the canal, and cauda equina nerve roots.

Symmetry and asymmetry: Cauda equina nerves are normally situated in a symmetrical position with half on the right and half on left sides of the spinal canal. Asymmetry means that some nerve roots have been displaced or shifted from their normal position due to a disease process.

Thickening: Cauda equina nerves have a rather standard thickness. Thickening or enlargement means the roots have edema, inflammation, and/or scarring

SELECTED BIBLIOGRAPHY

1. Addison T. The Constitutional and Local Effects of Disease of the Supra-Renal Capsules. Samuel Highley, London, 1855.

2. Aldrete JA. Arachnoiditis: The Silent Epidemic. Future Medical Pub, Mexico, 2003.

3. Francomano CA, Hakim AJ, Henderson LG, et al. Symptomatic: The Symptom-Based Handbook for Ehlers-Danlos Syndromes and Hypermobility Spectrum Disorders. Elsevier Amsterdam, 2024.

4. Javin D. Disjointed: Navigating the Diagnosis and Management of Hypermobile Ehlers-Danlos Syndrome and Hypermobile Spectrum Disorders. Hidden Stripes Pub San Francisco, CA, 2020.

5. Tennant F. Adhesive Arachnoiditis: An Old Disease Re-Emerges. Tennant Foundation, West Covina, CA, 2019.

REFERENCES

1. Aldrete JA. Suspecting and diagnosing arachnoiditis. *Pract Pain Mgt* 2006;16:74-87.
2. Anderson TL, Morris JM, Wald JT, et al. Imaging appearance of advanced chronic adhesive arachnoiditis: A retrospective review. *Am J Roentgenol* 2017;209:648-655.
3. Austin PJ, Moaleno-Taylor G. The neuro-immune balance in neuropathic pain: involvement of inflammatory immune cells, immune-like glial cells and cytokines. *J Neuroimmunol* 2010;229:26-50.
4. Beighton P, DePaepe A, Steinman B, et al. Ehlers-Danlos Syndrome: revised nosology. Villefranche 1997. *Am J Med Genet* 1998;77:33-37.
5. Bilello J, Tennant F. Patterns of chronic inflammation in extensively treated patients with arachnoiditis and chronic intractable pain. *Postgrad Med* 2016;92:1-5.
6. Bjornevik K, Cortese M, Healy BC, et al, et al. Longitudinal analysis reveals high prevalence of Epstein-Barr virus associated with multiple sclerosis. *Science* 2022;375:296-301.
7. Burcharth J, Rosenberg J. Gastrointestinal surgery and related complications in patients with Ehlers-Danlos Syndrome: a systemic review. *Dig Surg* 2012;29:349-357.
8. Byers PH, Murray ML. Heritable collagen disorders: the paradigm of the Ehlers-Danlos Syndrome. *J Invest Dermatol* 2012;132:6-11.
9. Carroll, MB. Hypermobility spectrum disorders: a review. *Rheumatol Immunol* Res 2023;4:60-68.
10. Castori M, Voermann NC. Neurological manifestations of "Ehlers-Danlos Syndromes. *Iran J of Neurol* 2014;13:190-208.
11. Cazzato D, Castori M, Lombardi R, et al. Small fiber neuropathy is a common feature of Ehlers-Danlos Syndrome. *Neurolgy* 2016;87:155-159.

12. Chan AC, Wilder-Smith E. Small fiber neuropathy: getting bigger! *Muscle Nerve* 2016;53:671-682.
13. Chang CW, Peng P. Failed back surgery syndrome. *Pain Med* 2011;12:577-606.
14. Chang DM, Chu SJ, Chen HC, et al. Dehydroepiandrosterone suppresses interleukin 10 synthesis in women with systemic lupus erythematosus. *Ann Rheum Dis* 2004;63:1623-1620.
15. Chiarelli N, Ritelli M, Zoppi N, et al. Cellular and molecular mechanisms in the pathogenesis of classical, vascular, and hypermobile Ehlers-Danlos Syndromes. *Genes* 2019;10:69-91.
16. Chopra P, Tinkle B, Hamonet C, et al. Pain management in the Ehlers-Danlos syndromes. *Am J Med Genet C Semin Med Genet* 2017;175C:212-219.
17. Danlos M. Un cas de cutis laxa avec tumeurs par contusion chronique des coudes et des genoux. *Bull Soc Franc Derm* Syph 1908;19:70-72.
18. Duan Y, et al. Immune cell infiltration and the genes associated with ligamentum flavum hypertrophy: identification and validation. Front Cell Dev Biol 2022;10:91478.
19. Ehlers E. Cutis laxa, niegung zu haemorrhaglen in der haut, lockerung mehrer artikulationen. *Derm Z* 1901;8:173-175.
20. Eisenberg E, Goldman R, Schlag-Eisenberg D, et al. Adhesive arachnoiditis following lumbar epidural steroid injections: A report of two cases and review of literature. *J Pain Research* 2019;12:513-518.
21. Fernandez A, Rozier BA, Vautey M, et al. Small fiber neuropathy in hypermobile Ehlers-Danlos Syndrome/hypermobility spectrum disorder. *J Intern Med* 2022;292:957-960.
22. Fine PG. Long-term consequences of chronic pain: mounting evidence for pain as a neurologic disease and parallels with other chronic disease states. *Pain Med* 2011;12:996-1004.

23. Gelse K, Poschi E, Aigmer T. Collagen structure, function, and biosynthesis. *Adv Drug Deliv Rev* 2003;55:1531-1546.
24. Grahame R. Joint hypermobility syndrome pain. *Curr Pain Headache Ret* 2009;13:427-433.
25. Grahame R. Heritable disorders of connective tissue. *Best Pract Res Clin Rheumatol* 2000;14:345-361.
26. Haensch CA, Tusch M, Katona L, et al. Small fiber neuropathy with cardiac denervation in postural tachycardia syndrome. *Muscle Nerve* 2014;50:956-961.
27. Hakim AJ, Grahame R. A simple questionnaire to detect hypermobility: an adjunct to the assessment of patients with diffuse musculoskeletal pain. *In J Clin Pract* 2003;57:163-166.
28. Hamonet C, Ducret L. Ehlers-Danlos, an unknown and disturbing syndrome, free comments. *Theranostics Brain, Spine, and Neurol Disord* 2017;2:555-591.
29. Harley JB, Chan X, Pujato M, et a. Transaction factors operate across disease loci, with EBNA2 implicated in autoimmunity. *Nat Genet* 2018;50:699-707.
30. Harrow T. Epstein-Barr virus could be a cause of multiple autoimmune disorders. *VA Research Currents* April 18, 2018.
31. Henderson FC, Austin C, Benzel E, et al. Neurological and spinal manifestations of the Ehlers-Danlos Syndromes. *Amer J Med Gen* 2017;175C195-211.
32. Horsley V. Chronic spinal meningitis: its differential diagnosis and surgical treatment. *Br J Med* 1909;1:513-517.
33. Houen G, Trier NH. Epstein-Barr virus and systemic autoimmune disease. *Front Immunol* 2020;11:1-13.
34. Huitsm E, DeVries J, Drent M. The small fiber neuropathy screening list: construction and cross validation in sarcoidosis. *Repair Med* 2011;105:95-100.
35. Hung AL, Lim M, Doshi TC. Targeting cytokines for treatment of neuropathic pain. *Scand J Pain* 2017;17:287-293.

36. Igharo D, Thiel JC, Rolke R, et al. Skin biopsy reveals generalized small fiber neuropathy in hypermobile Ehlers-Danlos syndromes. *Eur J Neurol* 2022;30:719-728.
37. Indari O, Tiwari D, Tanwar M, et al. Early biomolecular changes in brain microvascular endothelial cells under Epstein-Barr virus influence: A Raman microspectroscopic investigation. *Integr Biol* 2022;14:89-97.
38. Indari O, Jakhomola S, Pathak DK, et al. Comparative account of biomolecular changes post Epstein Barr virus infection of the neuronal and glial cells using Raman microspectroscopy. *ACS Chem Neurosci* 2022;13:1627-1637.
39. Jackson A, Isherwood I. Does degenerative disease of the lumbar spine cause arachnoiditis? A magnetic resonance study and review of the literature. *Brit J Radiology* 1994;67:840-847.
40. Jakhmola S, Jha HM. Glial cell response to Epstein Barr Virus infection: a plausible contribution to virus-associated inflammatory reactions in the brain. *Virology* 2021;559:182-195.
41. Javida E, Magnus T. Autoimmunity after ischemic stroke and brain injury. *Front Immunol* 2019;10:1-12.
42. Jones KJ. Gonadal steroids and neuronal regeneration: a therapeutic role. *Adv Neurol* 1993;59:227-240.
43. Kerr J. Epstein Barr Virus (EBV) reactivation and therapeutic inhibitors. *J Clin Pathol* 2019;0:1-8.
44. Kiefer, etal. Effects of dexamethasone on microglial activation in vitro. *J Neuroimmunology* 1991;34:99-108.
45. Kiguchi N, et al. Chemokines and cytokines in neuroinflammation leading to neuropathic pain. *Curr Opinion Pharmacol* 2012;12:55-61.
46. Kim ST, Brinjikii W, Lanzino G, et al. Neurovascular manifestations of connective tissue diseases: a review. *Intern Neuroradial* 2016;22:624-637.
47. Maier A, Kapfenberger R, Katano I, et al. Nonregional small fiber neuropathy in cases of autoimmune autonomic neuropathy. J Neurol 2022;269:6648-6654.

48. Malfait F, Francomano C, Byers P, et al. The 2017 international classification of the Ehlers-Danlos syndromes. *Am J Med Genet C Semin Med Genet* 2017;175:8-26.
49. Meisel C, Schwab JM, Prass K, et al. Central nervous system injury-induced immune deficiency syndrome. *Nat Rev Neurosci* 2005;6:775-786.
50. Mika J, Zychowska M, Popiolek-Barczy K, et al. Importance of glial activation in neuropathic pain. *Eur J Pharmacol* 2013;716:106-119.
51. Milligan ED, Watkins LR. Pathological and protective roles of glia in chronic pain. Nat Rev Neurosci 2009;10:23- 36.
52. Oaklander AL. Immunotherapy prospects for painful small fiber sensory neuropathies and gangliopathies. *Neurotherapeutics* 2016;13:108-117.
53. O'Callgan JP, SriranT, Miller DB. Defining "neuroinflammation". *Ann NY Acad Sci* 2008;1139:318-330.
54. Palmer S, Bailey S, Barker L, et al. The effectiveness of therapeutic exercise for joint hypermobility syndrome: a systemic review. *Physiotherapy* 2014;100:220-227.
55. Parenti V, Huda F, Richardson PK, et al. Lumbar arachnoiditis: Does imaging associate with clinical features? *Clin Neurol Neurosurg* 2020;192:105717.
56. Poscarello A, Provitera V, Lullo F, et al. Evidence of small fiber neuropathy in a patient with Ehlers-Danlos Syndrome, hypermobility type. *Clin Neurophysiol* 2016;127:1914-1916.
57. Prockop DJ, Kivirikko KI. Heritable diseases of collagen. *N Engl J Med* 1984;311:376-386.
58. Reddy DS. Neurosteroids: endogenous role in the human brain and therapeutic potentials. *Prog Brain Res* 2010;186:13-137.
59. Rodriguez LJG, Sandoval Sanchez V, Benavides Rodriguez D, et al. Paraplegia due to adhesive

arachnoiditis: a case report. *Act Ortop Mex* 2009;23:232-236.

60. Rombaut L, Scheper M, De Wandele J, et al. Chronic pain in patients with the hypermobility type of Ehlers-Danlos syndrome: Evidence for generalized hyperalgesia. *Clin Rheumatol* 2015;34:1121-1129.
61. Sacheti A, Szemere J, Bernstein B, et al. Chronic pain is a manifestation of the Ehlers-Danlos Syndrome. *J Pain Symptom Manage* 1997;14:88-93.
62. Saperstein DS. Small fiber neuropathy. *Neurol Clin* 2020;38:607-618.
63. Schievink WI, Gordon OK, Tourje J, et al. Connective tissue disorders with spontaneous spinal cerebrospinal fluid leaks and intracranial hypotension: a prospective study. *Neurosurgery* 2004;54:65-71.
64. Schremp FW, Katona I, Dugan I, et al. Reduced intraepidermal nerve fiber density in patients with REM sleep behavior disorder. *Parkinsonism Relat Disord* 2016;29:10-16.
65. Sene D. Small fiber neuropathy: diagnosis, causes, and treatment. *Joint Bone Spine* 2018;85:553-559.
66. Sevesto S, Merli P, Ruggier M, et al. Ehlers-Danlos Syndrome and neurological features: a review. *Childs Neuro Syst* 2011;27:365-371.
67. Takahashi H, Sugura T, Okazimo Y, et al. Inflammatory cytokines in the herniated disc of the lumbar spine. Spine 1996;21:218-224.
68. Voermans NC, Knoop H, Bleijinberg G, et al. Pain in Ehlers-Danlos Syndrome is common, severe, and associated with functional impairments. *J Pain Symptom Manage* 2010;40:370-378.
69. Wang L, Wang FS, Gershwin ME. Human autoimmune disease: a comprehensive update. *J Intern Med* 2015;278:369-395.
70. Weis J, Katona I, Muller-Newen, et al. Small fiber neuropathy in patients with ALS. *Neurology* 2011;76:2024-2029.

71. Whendon JM, Glassey D. Cerebrospinal fluid stasis and its clinical significance. *Altern Ther Health Med* 2009;15:54-60.
72. Yew KS , Kamps-Schmidt KA, Gorge R. Hypermobile Ehlers-Danlos Syndrome and hypermobility spectrum disorders. *Am Fam Physician* 2021;103:481-492.
73. Zang Y, Chee A, Shi P, et al. Intervertebral disc cells produce interleukins found in patients with back pain. *Am J Phys Med* 2016;95:407-415.
74. Zhang N, Zou Y, Jiang L, et al. Epstein Barr virus and neurologic diseases. *Front Mol Biosci* 2022;10:1-34.
75. Zhou Z, Rewari A, Shanthanna H. Management of chronic pain in Ehlers-Danlos syndrome. *Medicine (Baltimore)* 2018;97:45.
76. Zweiman B, Levinson AI. Immunologic aspects of neurological and neuromuscular diseases. *JAMA* 1992;268:2918-2922.

INDEX

OTHER BOOKS BY FOREST TENNANT

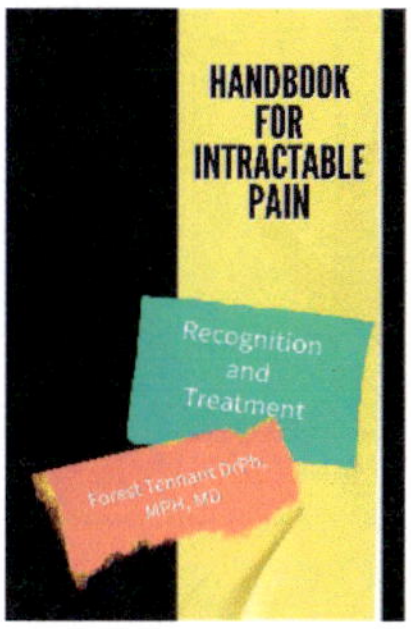

Handbook For Intractable Pain

ISBN:9781955934329
LOC:2023921074

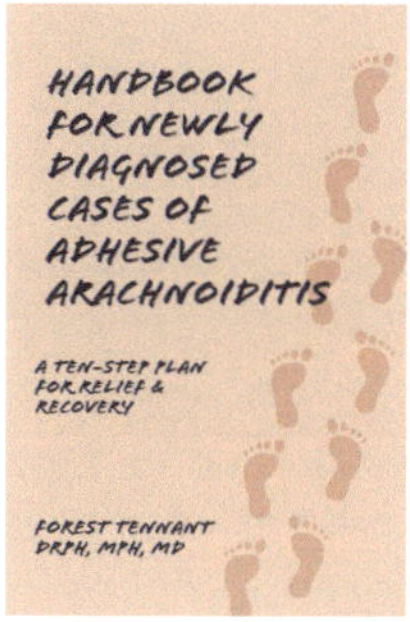

Handbook For Newly Diagnosed Cases of Adhesive Arachnoiditis

ISBN:9781955934244
LOC:2023908116

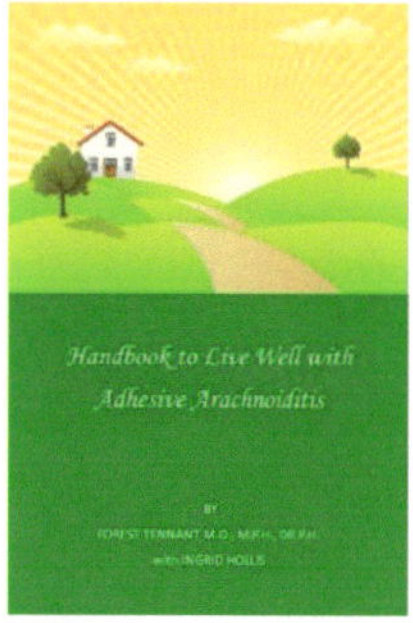

Handbook to Live Well with Adhesive Arachnoiditis

ISBN 978195934060
LOC: 2021912718

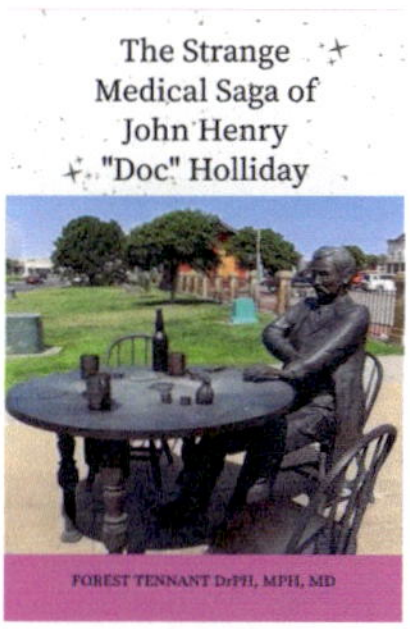

The Strange Medical Saga of "John Henry"

ISBN:9781955934275
LOC 2023913628

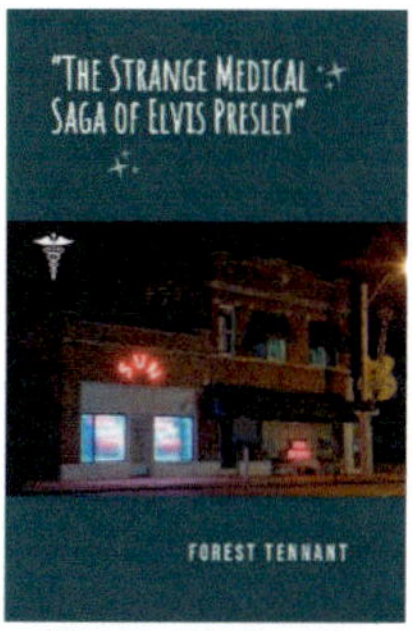

The Strange Medical Saga of Elvis Presley

ISBN: 9781955934008
LOC: 2021911718

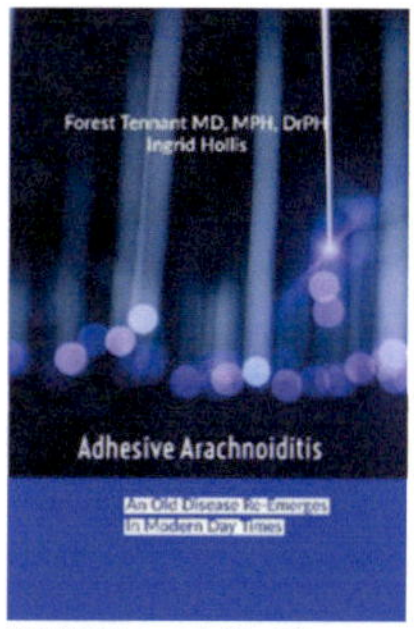

An Old Disease Re-Emerges in Modern Times

ISBN:9781955934039
LOC:2021912467

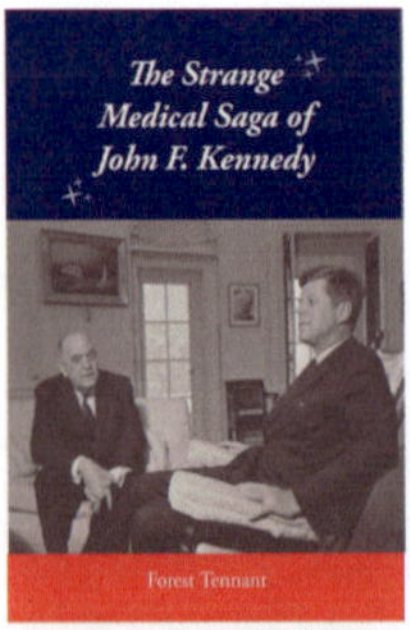

The Strange Medical Saga of JFK

ISBN:9781955934213
LOC:2023903440

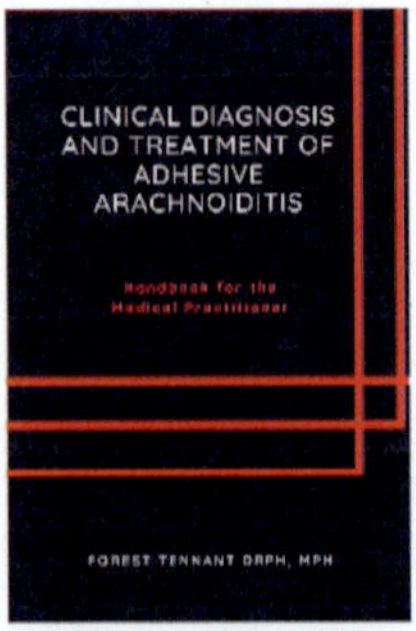

Clinical Diagnosis and Treatment of Adhesive Arachnoiditis

ISBN: 9781955934183
LOC: 2022907190

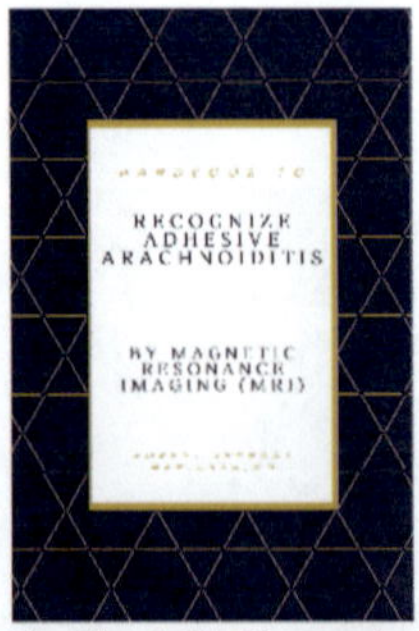

Handbook To Recognize Adhesive Arachnoiditis by Magnetic Resonance Imaging (MRI)

ISBN: 9781955934152
LOC: 2021925161

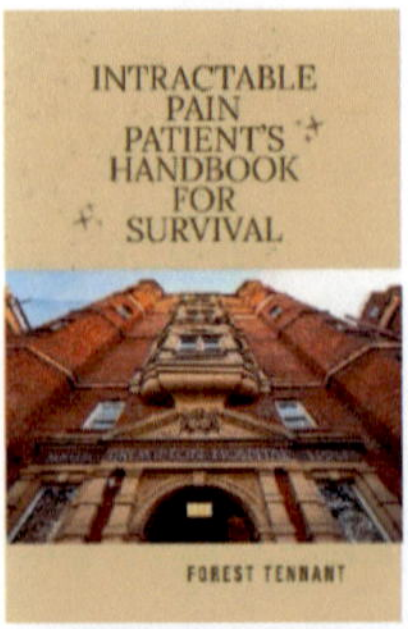

Intractable Pain Patients Handbook for Survival

ISBN: 9781955934121
LOC: 2021916464

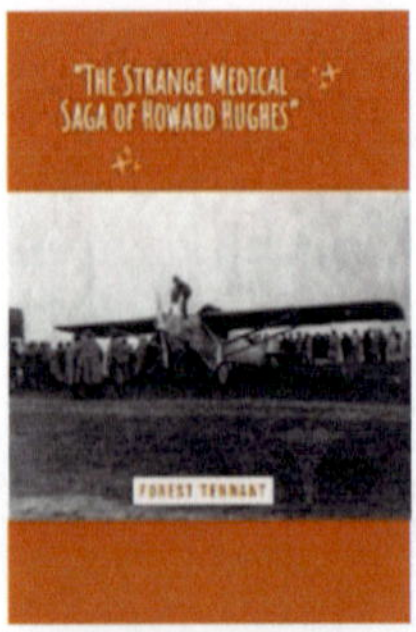

The Strange Medical Saga of Howard Hughes

ISBN: 9781955934091
LOC: 2021912855

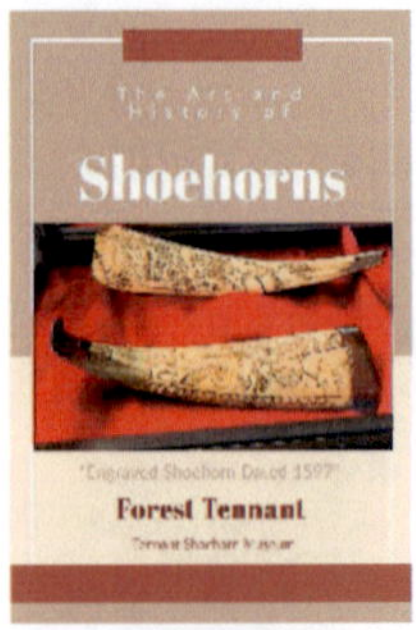

The Art and History of Shoehorns

ISBN:9781955934350
LOC:2024903219

Made in the USA
Columbia, SC
22 July 2026

4a261509-afe5-46a0-86f2-7dc7e66681a3R01